ELEVATE YOUR WELLBEING

Dearest Sandy,

Thankyou for the way you've elevated my wellbeing over the last 40 years with our beautiful friendship.

much love,

Heather xxx

14·2·19

ELEVATE YOUR WELLBEING

THE MOST INSPIRING WAY TO TAKE YOUR WELLBEING TO THE NEXT LEVEL

Foreword by Dr John Demartini
Human Behaviour Specialist, Educator & Teacher From 'The Secret'

Disclaimer

All the information, techniques, skills and concepts contained within this publication are of the nature of general comment only and are not in any way recommended as individual advice. The intent is to offer a variety of information to provide a wider range of choices now and in the future, recognising that we all have widely diverse circumstances and viewpoints.

Should any reader choose to make use of the information contained herein, this is their decision, and the contributors (and their companies), authors and publishers do not assume any responsibilities whatsoever under any condition or circumstances. It is recommended that the reader obtain their own independent advice.

First Edition 2018

National Library of Australia
Cataloguing-in-Publication entry:

Title: Elevate Your Wellbeing
ISBN(s): 9781925471342
Series: Elevate Books

Creator: Harvey, Benjamin J., author.
Other Authors:
Adelin, Deborah | Alexander, Jordan |Bolto, Tina |Chin, Irene |English, Bridget| Lam, Annie | McAlpine, Heather | Morrison, Kathy |Pitt, Gretchen | Zsolnai, Debbie

 A catalogue record for this book is available from the National Library of Australia

Published by Author Express
www.AuthorExpress.com
publish@authorexpress.com

Dedication

*To fellow learners wanting to take
their wellbeing to the next level. This
book is dedicated to you.*

Benjamin J Harvey and co-authors

elevate

Foreword by Dr John Demartini

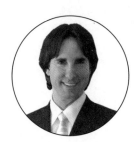

For over forty years, I've studied the art of wellness and the healing arts, particularly in relation to the mind-body connection. I have a background as a chiropractor, and I study the integration of psychology and philosophy.

In particular I've been involved in axiology, which is the study of worth and values. Every human being lives by a hierarchy of values, and no two people have the same ones. People's values, or priorities, are as unique to that individual as their fingerprints or eye retina. Because of this, people filter the world through their values and perceive situations.

Something that's of highest value is what you're inspired from within to do. No one needs to remind you to get up in the morning. You love doing it. On the other hand, you procrastinate on the lowest values and require outside motivation.

The hierarchy of these values also affects your physiology. In other words, how the body functions. How you perceive the world according to your values affects your cells, genetics and physical condition.

There's an underlying psychology of health conditions people have in their everyday lives. The body shows you signs and symptoms as feedback to point you in the direction and guide you to be your most congruent, authentic and inspired self in order to live your most fulfilled life. Basically, if you're not living according to your highest values, you're low on energy and have illness in the body. Hate and anger can run down the immune system. It's a well-known fact that anger, loss and stress can lead to cancer. Unbalanced emotions will lead to illness, and love and appreciation will lead you back to wellness.

Vitality in life is proportionate to your vision. You're in the highest vibration when you're living your authentic life. When you live according to your highest values, you're rewarded physiologically with increased energy.

Throughout this book you will find healers with various methodologies, all ultimately working to bring your body back to homeostasis. A therapist or healer who works from a space of love and gratitude of the heart and certainty and presence of mind, will affect a healing in anyone with whom he/she comes into contact. There's absolutely a place for their healing modalities and treatments, though it's important to realise that all true wellness starts in the mind and works through the heart.

In terms of health, I believe everyone should eat to live and not live to eat. Drink lots of water, and be grateful.

You can be a master of your destiny or a victim of your history. When you go to bed with gratitude, you wake up with inspiration. I'm certain that practicing gratitude will Elevate Your Wellbeing.

What I know for sure is that gratitude causes your heart to open and for love to flow, and love is the greatest healer in life.

Dr John F. Demartini
Human Behaviour Specialist
www.DrDemartini.com

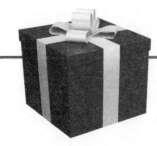

BONUS GIFT

The Elevate YOU
7 Day Transformation

Want to take the top 7 areas of your life to the next level?

There is ONE powerful 'Elevate Process' you can use immediately to improve Your Relationships, Health, Finances, Mindset and any other area of your life.

In this transformational 7 day online course, Benjamin J Harvey guides you through the 'Elevate Process' and how you can improve your life from the inside-out.

Normally valued at $295
Get FREE and instant access here:

www.elevatebooks.com/you

Life Rewards Action. Get started today!

Contents

"Giving yourself permission
to do what you love is the key to
elevating all areas of your life."

~ *Benjamin J Harvey*

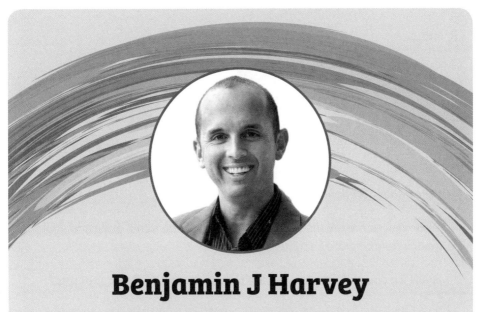

Benjamin J Harvey

Authentic Happiness

In his pursuit to assist people in finding the answers to life's most intriguing questions, Benjamin J Harvey has studied the psychology of empowerment for over ten years. Knowing that reading books like the Elevate series empowers people to bring their dreams into reality, Benjamin has been assisting thousands of people across the globe to empower themselves and live abundantly on purpose.

In 2009 he founded Authentic Education with business partner Cham Tang, to help people live a rich life. As a result, Authentic Education went on to achieve something that has never been done before in the history of personal development. They received the BRW Fast Starters Award in 2013 and then backed it up in 2015 by being named in the BRW Fast 100 as the thirty-eighth fastest-growing company in Australia.

Benjamin J Harvey

Authentic Happiness

What does "Wellbeing mean to you?"

Wellbeing to me means a state of wellness in the mind, body and soul leading to authentic happiness.

What do you tell people who say they just want to find happiness?

A lot of Dalai Lama's work is in relation to happiness, which is a common goal of the human race.

He understood happiness metaphysically but wanted to understand it scientifically as well, so he commissioned about two-hundred scientists of all different disciplines and asked them to go out into the scientific world and bring back the formula for happiness. After about a year or so worth of research, they all came back with a basic equation: $H=S+C+V$, with of course the "H" standing for happiness.

Now, "S" stands for your vibration set point. What these scientists discovered is that half of your current happiness is based on your memories, experiences, upbringing and traumas. They called it a set point, because what they worked out is that as you experience happiness, your vibration fluctuates up and down. The happier and more elated you are, the higher you vibrate, and the more depressed you are, the lower you vibrate.

Your set point for happiness on a scale of zero to one-hundred, vibrationally, might be eighty, but your resting set point might be forty, which means your happiest day would be equivalent to your most average day.

Everybody has a different set point of how much happiness they experience in a day. There are some people you meet who are just always happy and having a good time. You might have always wondered why, but it's just because their set point is higher. It would be fair to say that one of your neighbours' lowest days ever could be equivalent to your happiest day ever, due to their higher happy set point.

The good news is that you can work on your set point with certain techniques.

"C" stands for conditions of living and only makes up ten percent of your happiness.

So if you get that house by the beach you've always wanted, it still amounts to only ten percent of your happiness. This means that if you're unhappy before you got that house, you're going to still be unhappy afterwards.

That's why you meet people who look like they have it all on the surface, but they're miserable.

The sad thing is that people spend way more than ten percent of their time trying to increase their conditions of living. For instance, there's something called retail therapy, where a person goes to a shop and just buys stuff like shoes and clothing. What these scientists did is track the rush people get from this by looking at different neurotransmitters, which are molecules that jump across the synapse and only go into three small categories: the small peptide, which are fast-acting neurotransmitters that are excitatory and inhibitory signal responses, slow-acting small molecule neurotransmitters that modulate the way in which the system works and the large molecule, known as protein molecules, which are neuro-peptides that are even slower.

Large-moleculed neurotransmitters get affected by the blood brain barrier, or BBB, but the smaller molecules have an ability to pass around and move through it.

So by tracking the neurochemistry of these shoppers, the scientists observed that they were experiencing happiness, which was a release of endorphins, as well as oxytocin and other chemicals inside their brain, and that the releasing of these chemicals lasted a maximum of seventy-two hours.

This means the money you spend at that shop is a three-day drug. There are actual drugs that last longer.

A lot of people are trying to get happier by pouring money into a device that will only give them seventy-two hours worth of happiness. That's why if you can't manage your emotions, you won't be able to manage your money, because you'll just keep spending it.

So if you only get a ten percent chance of being happy from changing your living conditions, my advice is to not even bother working on that. Forget about the new suit and new shoes. If you're trying to achieve happiness this way, don't do it. There's no point to it. Zero.

The "V" stands for voluntary choices or actions made in the present moment and accounts for forty percent of your happiness. You have your set point, which is all of your past that determines half of how happy you are today. You have the shoes and new clothes you're wearing, which translates to ten percent of how happy you are. And the remaining forty percent of your happiness is governed by your voluntary choices and actions in the present moment.

What do they mean by that?

My favourite quote of all time is by Art Linkletter, who says, "Things turn out best for the people who make the best out of the way things turn out." What he means is that no matter what happens, if you make the best out of it, you're going to have the best life, but if you make the worst out of it, you'll have the worst life.

In certain forms of neurocommunication modalities, they class it as something called utilisation, where you use anything and everything to your advantage. So, let's say you walk out to your car to go to work and find someone has keyed it. You say, "Yes! New paint job!" Or you're travelling through Paris, and someone takes your backpack. Your first response is, "That thing was so heavy." Even if you're standing in an empty house because someone has robbed you, your reaction could be, "My old couch was so worn out and hurt my back, and now I can get a new one!" No matter what life throws at you, it doesn't have to get you down.

Now, these people aren't ignorant to the downside. They realise all their stuff has been stolen. They get that. But what they also understand is that it's an instant opportunity to feel grateful.

The people that are able to do this actually transform the amygdala response, which is the split-second reaction to what life's chucking at you. They rewire how they respond to whatever is responsible for their fears and anxieties. They know it's there, but they just don't focus on it. (People refer to this space between stimulus and response as the gap.)

What these scientific researchers also did was put people under Electrocardiograph (ECG) machines that measure heart cycles, brain cycles, and movement, as well as magnetic resonance imaging (MRI) machine to track liquid movement, and showed them negative, neutral and positive images while monitoring their brain behaviour.

What they found is that happy people dwelled longer on the happy image than they did on the negative ones. They made a conscious, voluntary choice to save the happy images longer. When a happy person walks down the street, they do see all of the crap, but they focus on it for less time than the people who are unhappy. They have pre conditioned their brain to look for things to be happy about.

Is it important to always remain positive in order to be authentically happy?

I once spoke with a man who was in Risk Management and said his job was to look at everything that could go wrong, and he worried about what that meant for his attitude.

What I told him is that just because you're looking at everything that can go wrong doesn't mean you have a bad attitude. I want to make that distinction. Those who refuse to look at the downside live in a fantasy. A lot of people don't realise that if they refuse to look at the downside of life, the risk is great they'll never get to their destination. It'll be two steps forward, ten steps back. Seeing what can go wrong doesn't mean you're being negative. It means you're strategic. It means you're intelligent. However, those who only look at the downside and say, "Oh my goodness, we're doomed," aren't being any more realistic. It only indicates a bad attitude. It's those who say, "How do we overcome it?" who are the ones with a great attitude.

A lot of people say, "That guy at work, he's so negative," or, "She's so negative. She always points out what goes wrong," but without that person you might not see the downside. It's those who point out everything that could go wrong but do nothing about it who have a bad attitude. It's an important distinction.

What is The Gap?

Voluntary choice has a huge impact on your happiness. The problem is, you don't typically have a lot of time between what life throws at you and how you respond to that.

But there's a way you can have a voluntary choice. Please refer to the simple diagram below.

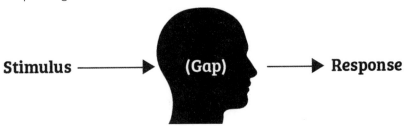

Stimulus ⟶ **(Gap)** ⟶ **Response**

As you can see, there's point one, which is the stimulus, and point two is the response. So in point one, you yell at someone, and in point two they yell back. The gap between you yelling at someone and them getting angry and yelling back equals how much voluntary choice you have.

Now in life, it's nanoseconds. For instance, you get cut off, and you honk your horn. You didn't choose this response. There was no volunteering. It was a nanosecond. The reason is because fifty percent of your programming said, "That person was rude. Honk your horn." You didn't make a choice about your reaction.

When you speak to yogis, they will talk about this thing called the gap. You want to meditate? Enter the gap. You want to be spiritual? Enter the gap. You want to have a better life? Enter the gap.

The gap is the distance between stimulus and response. The bigger the gap, the greater your voluntary choice; the smaller the gap, the less your voluntary choice. That's it. If you want to have a happier life, all you have to do is extend the gap between these two points.

Is there a way to extend The Gap?

Extending the gap requires practice that comes in the form of meditation. There are many different meditating techniques, and none are better or worse than the others. All I'm interested in, is if the meditation works. That's the most important thing.

I meet a lot of people who've been meditating for years, and there's still no gap between stimulus and response. None. They'll say, "Well, I've been meditating for forty years, and I had this incredible ... Shut up! I'm freaking talking!" "Anyway, I'm so Zen. I'm just totally into peace." It's like, why do they bother meditating? It's obviously not working. Stop it.

Remember, it's not that you know so much, it's that you know so much that isn't so. Most people who think they're meditating are not meditating. They're doing guided imagination healing (GIH), which is not meditation. That doesn't assist you in having a gap between stimulus and response. It assists you in becoming relaxed, yes, but it doesn't assist you in creating the gap.

A lot of people listen to these CDs of a river running down pebbles as they're told they're sitting in a forest where wise people come around with hoods on and shine their light on them before they float up and fly around. I love those. I do them all the time, but I'm not ignorant enough to believe that's meditation, because if this is all you do, I hate to tell you, but your gap is only getting smaller.

This is because guided imagery healing makes you super aware of everything. Now, if you're way more aware of everything around you, you're getting triggered way more than everybody else. This means if you don't match awareness with balance, you're in all sorts of trouble.

Twenty years later, after all this supposed meditation, these people aren't any more emotionally in control than they were before. That's because to make it more marketable, they called it guided meditation, when it was really guided imagery healing.

If all you do is awareness-based activities, you'll be more agitated than ever before and make connections that don't exist, while not understanding why the other person isn't making them as well.

Or maybe you study a different type of meditation, where it's all about balance. You stare at a candle and don't move for hours. This method will make you fully balanced, but you'll have no awareness.

I've had many different meditation teachers. One of them, a gentleman by the name of S.N. Goenkam who does *Vipassana* meditation, described it like wings of a butterfly. He says they have to be equal in strength and size, or they can't fly. These wings are balance and awareness. So if you only work on your balance, your gap is too big to be aware of anything, and if all you concentrate on is awareness, your gap is too small to be attuned to anything.

The perfect balance of these two is meditation. A lot of people use guided imagery for escapism, because for that one hour while they're down at their running nook, they're escaping life, and they feel better, but that doesn't transform any of the neurological pathways in the mind to help deal with that crappy stuff when the guided imagination process is over. They're not building and expanding their gap.

There's a saying that a mind once stretched, can never go back to its original dimensions. Or, as Wayne Dyer used to say, "A set of Speedos once stretched, will never go back to their original dimensions."

So you learn a little bit of information and expand your mind, and then maybe you pick up a book, apply a little bit and expand your mind. Then you attend a seminar and expand it even more. You start off with a small consciousness and keep stretching it until your world gets pretty big, and you'll start to believe you have a pretty expansive consciousness.

So meditation puts a massive gap between the stimulus and how you choose to respond. The bigger the gap, the more you get to voluntarily choose how you feel, which probably wouldn't include resentment, disgust, furiousness or complete body-numbing anger.

But if you don't have a gap, you can't make the choice.

How does meditation work?

I want to explain meditation to you in a way that you'll get it, because a lot of people meditate but don't know what they're doing, so they aren't really meditating.

The beautiful thing about meditation is that there's no delay. It's the most instantly gratifying technique you can do on planet Earth, and the benefits last, on average, about twenty-four hours.

Meditators activate the executive function, which is when eight specific functions in the brain all switch on at once to help you manifest what you want as if out of thin air. They are: impulse control, organisation, self-monitoring, emotional control, flexibility, working memory, task initiation and planning and prioritisation.

The reason meditators seem to have ESP and the ability to synchronistically put things together and perceive events before they happen, is due to a heightened executive function. It looks magical, but it's just the brain doing what it's meant to be doing.

How can meditation be used to slow the aging process?

Mystical things do occur when you meditate, but if you forget about this for a second and just look at meditation in a scientific light, you'll see something miraculous. I've done research at the anti-aging clinic where they do extensive research on what stops people from aging.

Basically there are three chemicals in the body that if you know how to regulate, increase or reduce them, you can age way more slowly than everybody else.

1. DHEA

DHEA is the precursor to all hormones in the body. New research is showing that DHEA is your body's natural steroid. You turn it on, and it does what it's meant to do. If you have a reduction in DHEA inside your system, you'll actually experience things like chronic fatigue syndrome.

The Anti-Aging Clinic Association of America has discovered that when someone meditates, they can increase DHEA anywhere from 87 to 380 percent that day. That's pretty amazing. DHEA stops you from aging and assists a whole lot of body functions to slow down the aging process.

2. Melatonin

The other thing that happens when you meditate is that you produce a substance called melatonin. When you're meditating, melatonin production can increase anywhere from 100 to 250 percent, which means you feel more rested and don't have to sleep as much, because you don't feel as lethargic.

Now if you produce melatonin while you're meditating, it means the body perceives it's resting more than it is, and if that's the case, you don't age as much. Because if you want to quicken the aging process, just stop sleeping as much. Reduce your sleeping to two hours a night and watch how fast you age. You can look in the mirror and see it happen. If you meditate and increase that melatonin, and trick the system into believing it's sleeping more than it is, then it has an impact on aging.

3. Cortisol

Cortisol is great to have in your system. A lot of people say you need to get rid of it, it, but you don't. You need cortisol. You just don't need a lot of it, and most people have more than they need. Cortisol does affect blood pressure and a whole range of activities, but generally when you get stressed out, your cortisol levels increase.

A twenty-minute meditation in the morning can reduce cortisol production by 47 percent. You can nearly halve your cortisol by meditating.

Here's another interesting fact. They biologically tested meditators and non-meditators and found that a non-meditator on average is about two to three years older than their biological age, while a meditator is twelve years *younger* than their biological age.

There's no reason left not to meditate. It doesn't even have to be a spiritual practice if you don't want it to be. It's just a way of getting more out of your brain and your body.

How does meditation affect the brain cycle?

If you were hooked up to an EEG machine and observed doing different behaviours, you would discover that your brain has different cycles.

If you've ever had a song stuck in your head, you should know the only way to get it out is to go to sleep. This is because as you awaken, your head is changing the cycles per second at which it's spinning.

As you're slowly waking up, your brain gets faster and faster. This is when you're in beta, which are high frequency, low amplitude brain waves that are involved in conscious thought, logical thinking, and tend to have a stimulating affect. Having the right amount allows you to focus and complete tasks easily. Alpha waves bridge the gap between your conscious thinking and subconscious mind, or the beta and theta. They help calm you down when necessary and promote feelings of deep relaxation.

So when you first wake up in the morning, instead of getting out of bed, just hold your posture and meditate for five minutes; don't move a muscle, even when your nose starts itching or your knee feels like it's going to explode and smash into a billion pieces. No matter what stimulus your body throws at you, don't respond. This is how your body will understand you're in control of it.

After a couple of days of doing this, the body will work out that unless the mind says you can do it, you can't do it. If you can sit there without moving and not scratch your nose for five minutes, what that equates to is a five-minute gap getting stuck in your head for the rest of the day. This means when someone comes up to you at work and metaphorically makes your nose itch, you don't scratch it. You just sit there and observe them. It's a nice sensation like a subtle vibration. And if you can sit there for twenty minutes without moving, that's a twenty-minute gap you can leverage all day long.

If you get this gap in your mind, you will realise that you're so much more balanced, even if you just put a two or three-minute gap in there, it will last all day. It's the most magnificent thing.

People reference time by liquid moving through their mind and body. If your brain wave speeds slow down or speed up, that reference of time gets warped quite significantly. When you first start meditating, set a timer or two, because you'll think it was five minutes, when it was twenty minutes. Or you'll think it was twenty minutes, and it'll be two minutes.

But after months, if not years, of meditation, your brain will never slow down again, and you'll be able to meditate exactly twenty minutes to the second. From the time you start meditating, your brain cycle is going to rise up and sit right on forty cycles per second, which is the ultimate speed the brain can travel so as to have every single function you ever want, running at its absolute prime. It's the most bizarre phenomena.

Meditation should be practised for enough time to get the maximum enjoyment from life and not a minute more, because if you get trapped in these deep, long sits, you might be using it as a form of escapism.

The purpose of morning meditation is not reacting. If you don't react, you've created a gap that lasts all day long. But if you wake up the next day and you don't do it again, the gap's gone. It's only there when you stick it in your head first thing in the morning.

Is there any particular method of meditation that's better than others? Do they need a special room or a particular kind of lighting?

Meditation is easy to do. There are no tricks to it. It's one of the most basic behaviours any human being can get good at.

First thing you want to do in the morning is trap a gap in your mind. You know what's easier than getting out of bed? Staying in bed. If you want to learn how to meditate, just don't get out of bed. There are people who say, "I have this special meditation room with a meditation cushion and my meditation incense with my meditation music," but all of that just stands for roadblock, roadblock, roadblock. My advice is to just meditate in bed, but not lying down. Once you become proficient at it, you can get your meditation room, but start in bed, because it'll just be an easier way of doing it.

There are only three real principles to meditation.

▶ **Principle One: stay still**

Not scratching your nose is a metaphor for life. If you sit there for five minutes with the itchiest nose ever and don't scratch it, you've now sacrificed the animal at the altar. I'm not talking about lambs and sheep but the hindbrain. It's about sacrificing, being a slave to this thing that wants to eat your nose and tell it that you're the master of it. And you do that through meditation.

Once you can sacrifice the animalistic nature of your brain, you control it, so stay still.

▸ **Principle Two: breathe naturally**

If your breathing is shallow, let it be shallow. If it's heavy, let it be heavy. Just don't change it. There are people who when they meditate, count their inhale for a count of five, hold it for a count of five, and then exhale for a count of five. If you're doing that, it's perfectly fine, it's just not meditating. It's counting breaths. I'm not disparaging it, because it's a great yogi practice. But again, it's not meditating. It's breath work.

So when you meditate, don't count your breaths. Don't change your breath. Because if you're doing that, you're reacting to life as opposed to allowing it to be as it is.

▸ **Principle Three: focus on the breath**

Just focus on your breath. If your mind wanders off, which is invariably going to happen, just bring it back to the breath. You may even go five minutes before you realise you haven't been focusing on it.

People treat meditation aggressively. They think to themselves, *Come on, brain. Back to the breath, man. I told you what to do. What are you thinking?* Well, that's not going to help you reach a state of inner peace. The second you realise you're not focusing on your breath, just imagine it as your best friend, and say, *Hey, best friend. Come on back to the breath. Yeah, it's okay. I know you have lots on your mind. It doesn't matter. Back to the breath, and forget about it.* Then when two seconds later it wanders off again, say, *Hey, come on back to the breath. Yeah, I know you've done it forty times already, but just come back again.*

You need to have infinite patience with bringing it back to the breath. You can't say that after ten times that you're going to be really pissed off. You can't do that. No matter how many times it wanders off, gently bring it back.

Is there a good meditation exercise to put all of these into practice?

Yes. Here are a few things to know before you begin.

1. Sit perfectly still with your feet flat on the floor and don't cross anything. This position is just a better way of getting energy flow for other practices you can do later on.

    If you choose to sit on the floor, cross your legs, but don't do full lotus. In the Western world, our hips and joints weren't designed for it. However, if you're easily able to do lotus, then go ahead and do it.

2. Do anything you want with your hands. You can interlock them or put them palms down or up. Just don't hold a position with your arms out and fingertips touching, so no yoga mudras, because then you have to consciously make sure your fingertips are touching, and then if you don't put effort into it, they open up.

    Just interlock them and put them in your lap, so that way you know they're not going to move anywhere.

3. Focus on the breath and breathe naturally. If your mind wanders, bring it back.

Elevate Your Wellbeing

If your nostrils are clear, breathe through your nostrils. It's the way you were designed as a species. You were never, ever meant to breathe through your mouth. You're meant to eat with your mouth. However, if your nose is blocked, then just breathe through your mouth.

4. If you're breathing through your nose, focus on the area just in the sort of triangle around your nostrils above your upper lip. The sensation of the breath blows across the top of your lip, adding mouth sensation on the lips. If you're breathing through your mouth, focus on the sensation of the breath crossing your lips.

5. Any time you get lost, gently bring it back.

    Here's the meditation. It's a pretty easy process. I'm not trying to replace your practice at all, but just try this technique and note the differences. Doing your own research is the most important thing. If meditation works, it works. It doesn't matter how you do it. There are many paths to the top of the mountain, and the view is always going to be the same.

Now, meditate for as long as you can at step 6. It can be 5 mins, 8 mins, or longer; the better you get at this, you will need to start setting your alarm. When you are ready to come out of the meditation, start from step 7 onwards. It is a really nice way to end the meditation.

1. Make sure your feet are flat on the floor, and gently close your eyes.

2. If you have to do one last little wriggle, go ahead and make that adjustment. Get it out of your system before sitting perfectly still.

3. Set the intention that you are a stone-chiselled statue. Don't move anything. Don't twitch a shoulder. Don't move a finger. Don't wriggle a toe, nothing. No matter what your body tells

you it wants to do, don't move your body. Just allow yourself to meditate.

4. Allow yourself to breathe naturally. Focus on your breath, and observe whatever it's doing. If your breath is shallow, let it be shallow. If it's deep, let it be deep.

5. Focus all of your awareness and attention on your breath. Observe it going in and out of the body, while not moving a single muscle. If something itches, do not scratch it. Do not be tricked by the body. No matter what the sensation, don't move a muscle. It's time to retrain the body, so it knows you control it, not the other way around.

6. If for any reason your mind begins to wander, gently bring it back. You are bound to be successful. You are destined to be successful. Sitting still, breathing naturally.

7. Take a nice, relaxing, deep breath and do a full-body smile. Imagine or pretend that out of the soles of your feet, you're beaming this incredibly vibrant smile. Just imagine the biggest smile you can possibly do with your feet.

8. Allow that smile to work its way up your legs, your shins, and to your calves.

9. Smile out of your knees; a big, bright, golden smile.

10. As you smile out of your feet and knees, allow that joy to work its way up through your thighs until you start to smile out of your hips.

11. Allow that smile to work its way up through your abdomen, the small of your back and out of your belly.

12. As that smile works its way up, imagine smiling out of your palms; this warm, joyous smile.

13. Allow that smile to work its way up your arms until you're smiling out of your elbows.

14. Then allow that smile to work its way up into your shoulders, until you're smiling out of your shoulders.

15. Now your chest is opening up. Smile from the centre of your heart out into the room. Just fill the room up with warmth, joy and love from your smile.

16. Now smile out of your back. Allow it to work its way up from the soles of your feet and up through your shins, your knees, your thighs, hips, and palms. That smile is working up through your chest and opening up your heart before working up into your shoulders.

17. Allow that smile to make its way up your neck and push through onto your face to fully express itself completely out to the world.

18. Allow your smile to travel up to the top of your head, so that every single cell in your entire being is smiling from the top of your head to the tips of your toes and all the way out through your fingertips.

19. With that nice, big smile on your face, take a relaxing deep breath in, and as you exhale, try to extend that smile above you by reaching your arms up towards the roof and then gently reach down towards the ground, just a little bit of a stretch. Then just slowly come back into an upright position.

20. Now wiggle your fingers and toes while keeping that nice big smile all the way through your body and on your face, and gently open your eyes. Keep wiggling your toes and fingers with a nice big smile on your face.

This meditation should last you for an entire day.

How does meditation lead to top-down management?

If you've seen the move *The Matrix*, you might have been led to believe that Neo is an anagram for (the) One. That's the biggest trick the movie played on you, because Neo isn't an anagram. It's actually referring to what Paul D. MacLean refers to as the neocortex, which is involved in higher functions such as sensory perception, initiation of motor commands, spatial reasoning, conscious thought, and language. What they're saying in *The Matrix*, is that when you elevate into the neocortex, you do something called top-down management, which means you govern the rest of the system. Bottom-up management is where you're just reacting to everything that happens.

The neocortex tells the entire system what it does or doesn't do. When you meditate, you now govern the matrix. The whole movie was a metaphor. It's a documentary about the brainstem and how you travel through it to get to the neocortex at the centre to override the entire matrix.

In the film, you'll see they're battling with instincts. They're moving up into imagination. Then they meet the architect, the intelligence, and Neo breaks through and becomes Neo.

What they explained in that film is that you can override the entire system. What's happening at a metaphysical, or even scientific level, is that you can learn exactly how to do those processes. You can do this through meditation.

Because what happens until you start living top down, you do what seems to be natural. If you're walking down the street at three in the morning and hear a loud sound behind you, your body gets into defence mechanism. This is checkpoint one, which is your instincts. Then you turn to see what it is, which is checkpoint two, the realm of imagination. You pattern match the image and see it's cats, so you go on to checkpoint three, intelligence, and ask yourself why cats are out there.

You go through these checkpoints whenever someone startles you. You're never going to be walking down the street at three in the morning, hear a loud sound and think to yourself, *Why are there cats?* It defies logic. That's why few people ever get to become Neo and live top-down. It defies all of the logical programming you think you've been given.

If you can go through life doing meaningful work without anything throwing you off course, you will live true to your mission. There'll be no distraction. That's from the neocortex, down the brainstem, and into the heart, the soul and the third eye. Now you're experiencing authentic living. That's really the epitome of authenticity.

How does meditation and brainwaves relate to trauma?

Some people's brainwaves go down when meditating instead of up. This is Delta Meditation. It happens from time to time. The reason for it, is because when you experience major trauma and spend most of your time in beta mode, if you get traumatised, to protect yourself, you spike down as low as you can go and store the trauma down there. Because if all your traumas in life were stored at this higher frequency, you couldn't operate.

When you first start meditating, the brain and the body say, "All right. You're meditating. You're getting control. You're not scratching your nose. You're not moving your legs. If you're in that level of control, we may as well start some healing now." Then it drops you down to where all of these traumas are, and starts releasing them out of the body. But it only does that once it realises you're not moving and are in control.

For the first couple of months you spend meditating, you'll actually start dipping down into all of these traumas, and sometimes you'll finish a meditation with quite a lot of aggression in the body. That's fine. Don't judge it. Just get on with your day. After a while of dipping down and picking up all of these traumas, there will be none left. You'll close your eyes to meditate and go straight up to gamma. But until you clear out all the stuff at those lower brainwave frequencies, you'll always dip down when you meditate. As you clear it out, you stop going for it.

That's why in a car accident, the whole world slows down. You're dipping to a lower frequency to store the memory as low as you can, so that it doesn't affect your waking state. That's how cool the brain is. It knows how to protect itself.

However, if you watch the accident take place, everything speeds up. This is because you're alert and in gamma. You're solving problems as fast as you can. You don't see an accident and slow down to theta before going over to help. You're on. Your brain is firing. It's working out solutions to help in any way possible. A lot of people think meditation is slowing you down, but it's only slowing down to clear the junk out. Once the junk's gone, your brain just does what it's meant to do at the optimum frequency of forty cycles per second.

Can you explain your program Prosper From Your Passion?

We have a one-day event called Prosper from your Passion where we teach a whole bunch of our business courses. I talk about personal development and three programs that specifically relate to creating major turning points around your ability to coach yourself, automate your success, and be exquisite at creating real wealth in your life.

There's an entire division of our company that train business people who want to make a difference. We work with only nine categories of business people:

- Coach

- Facilitator

- Consultant

- Seminar leader

- Keynote presenter

- Group coach

- Author

- Online educator

- Digital product creator

What we do when we start a program like this, is that we have people in our office who are course advisors. They advise people on the next steps to take either with their organisation or within other organisations. Our course advisors then block out a whole bunch of their calendar, so they can allocate some time to you. Basically, these course advisors are people who themselves have done our business programs and had a chat with our course advisors, received some great advice and strategies, and took the next step. Basically, these are some people who wanted to make a difference, so they took that next step.

Some people who've taken the course have been awarded the Telstra Small Business Award. One woman now gets paid to go on cruise ships to talk about time management.

The course advisors will help you align their passions, such as unpacking your masterpiece, learning how to create content, designing and positioning a brand to attract more people to your message, getting more clients or creating marketing campaigns. They can also help if you want to write courses, workshops or books.

Basically, the advisors run you through a series of eleven questions in order to clarify exactly where you are in the process of getting your business started, doing what you love, making a difference and transforming people's lives via your message and your mission. And from there, they give you strategic advice about the next steps to take.

 To discover more about how *Ben* can help you *Elevate Your Wellbeing,* simply visit www.elevatebooks.com/wellbeing

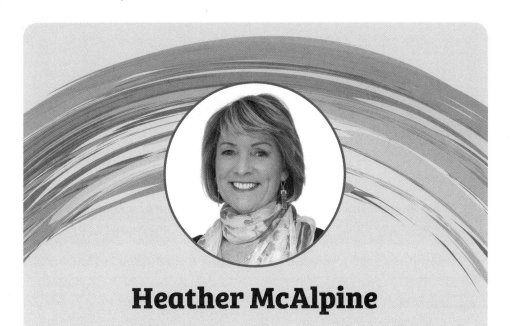

Heather McAlpine
Freedom Through Forgiveness

Heather McAlpine is a couples and family therapist, consultant and counselling supervisor. She's also an international speaker and presenter, was awarded the Winston Churchill Fellowship, has taught postgraduate and undergraduate students and was a Clinical Coordinator for Relationships Australia.

Throughout her over thirty-year career in counselling couples, Heather has enabled people to unleash their potential, so they can have fulfilling, vibrant and long-lasting relationships. She and her husband John are chair and trainer couple for Better Marriages Australia and run Couple Getaways.

Building on the theme of forgiveness, Heather has developed 'The Power of Apology', a popular two-day seminar that enables participants to enjoy the present by healing their past.

In her spare time, Heather enjoys long-distance cycling sustained by dark chocolate!

Heather McAlpine

Freedom Through Forgiveness

What inspired you to devote so much of your time as a relationship therapist and educator to the area of apologies and forgiveness?

A lot of my work involves enabling people to find resources within themselves, so they can restore their relationships and sometimes rebuild, from scratch, a brand-new one on a firmer foundation.

Reconciliations, big and small, are a major part of life. Just being human means stuffing up from time to time, so life is full of apology situations.

But often people find it difficult to apologise. Elton John sure was right when he sang, "Sorry seems to be the hardest word". Some people may find it easy to say the word "sorry", but even then, it often fails to have any positive impact.

Ten years ago, I received what I call a 'pseudo-apology' from someone who'd wounded me deeply.

At the beginning of the call when I asked, "How are you?" his response was, "Great day. Couldn't be better. Sorry if you're hurt...don't want to discuss it further". His words came across as trite and condescending, with no responsibility taken for the damage he'd caused.

I was later made a scapegoat, which added insult to injury. If I'd accepted the pseudo-apology, I would have been sucked into his world, joining him in his own denial, while pretending the issue had been resolved. It just would have made matters worse. Despite there being no request for forgiveness or acknowledgement of wrongdoing, I inwardly tried to forgive this person and pondered the complexity, confusion and chaos that unresolved issues can cause in relationships.

After facilitating countless relationship education programs, I became aware of a major gap in this field in regard to repairing relationship problems. Though I'd had the privilege of learning from the gurus in my profession through a Winston Churchill Fellowship that took me to the US and UK, I found few programs that focussed on enlightenment and healing as a way to free people from their past. It made me wonder how we could be more proactive in creating a therapeutic education model, as opposed to waiting until a person realised they needed counselling.

I became passionate about contributing in this area and designed a two-day program on inner healing that focussed on forgiving loved ones when core attitudes and actions cut into the soul and created deep wounds.

So, you put your passion into action. Who are you reaching with these programs?

Initially, I designed the *Power of Apology* program for those in the helping professions, but now I've opened it up to people in any profession. My aim is to enable everyone to appreciate the present by healing the past.

What part do genuine apologies and forgiveness play in truly healing the past?

I believe they're vital. It's not just the act of forgiving others, but forgiving yourself as well. People might have differing opinions as to how to apologise, or the importance of forgiveness, but the common ground lies in a deep desire for connection...the process of building emotional intimacy.

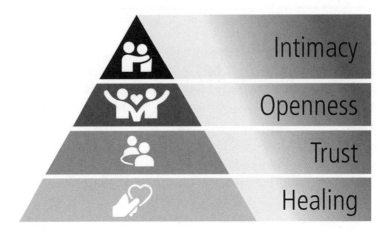

Intimacy is your destination, but it depends upon your willingness to remain **open**.

Openness enhances intimacy, but the degree to which you're open depends on your level of **trust**.

Trust is built on your ability to **heal past hurts.**

How does someone go about healing their past?

Unresolved, un-forgiven conflicts can pull you down and eat away at your soul, but the wonderful thing about close relationships is that by acknowledging you're on the same side, you can work together to heal your hurts.

Facing and resolving conflict, and forgiving those for whom you feel resentment and bitterness, are vital parts of the healing process. But it's not easy. Maybe you weren't raised in a family that encouraged self-awareness, so exploring what's underneath your anger can be a foreign concept.

Elevate Your Wellbeing

One way to discover your underlying feelings is to contain your anger and look deeper. Taking the time to explore and then express what's underneath it becomes a gift to yourself *and* your relationships.

Anger can arise from a multitude of feelings such as hurt, fear, shame, guilt, and humiliation, as well as feeling ignored, powerless and taken for granted. Other contributing factors could be underlying feelings of rejection or abandonment, as well as traumas from past life events.

The consequences from these traumas can be paramount.

Unhelpful attitudes and beliefs you may have picked up from childhood can re-emerge and stay, like an uninvited guest, even though they don't necessarily serve you well anymore. Although it's most likely your parents would have done the best they could with the resources they had at the time, you may have had some ongoing negative experiences. For example:

- ▸ If you weren't nurtured or made to feel special and significant as a child, you will crave the chance to be nurtured or feel significant as an adult.

- ▸ If you were deeply wounded through rejection, you will grow up with a filter of disapproval.

- ▸ If you were rejected through shame, it means you grow up living through a filter of guilt.

- ▸ If you were rejected through criticism, it means you grow up living through a filter of criticising others and always finding fault. This thought may seem gruesome, but getting rejected as a child could cause you to walk into a crowded room and believe everyone thinks you're no good.

On the other hand:

- ▸ Growing up with encouragement means you're more likely to feel worthwhile as an adult.

- ▸ Being raised with acceptance and approval means you'll tend to like yourself later in life.

- ▸ Growing up in a nurturing environment with healthy friendships will most likely translate to finding love in the world.

No matter how you were raised, you *can* take major steps towards inner healing.

In my Power of Apology couple programs, I enable couples to help each other towards inner healing as they use the resource of the relationship to set the scene for openness, vulnerability and growth.

But as individuals, everyone needs to take responsibility for their own personal development before expecting any real healing or growth to spring up within their relationships.

Why do past traumas or experiences have such a huge impact, even twenty years down the track?

Have you ever wondered why small, seemingly insignificant triggers can lead to unexpected and intense reactions? You may say to yourself, *Where did that come from?* Basic unconscious hurts, whether from a past partner or someone from your childhood, and can generate a huge angry reaction above and beyond the issue you're experiencing.

In terms of normal physical allergies, you could have a trigger that leads to an acute or even life-threatening reaction. As an example:

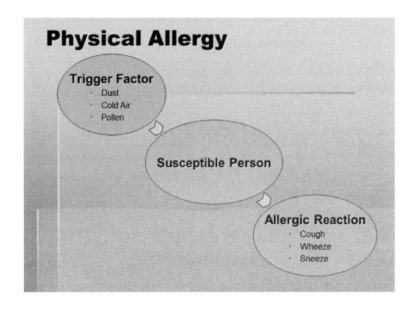

But you can also develop an emotional allergy and have an unexpected overreaction triggered by a past hurt.

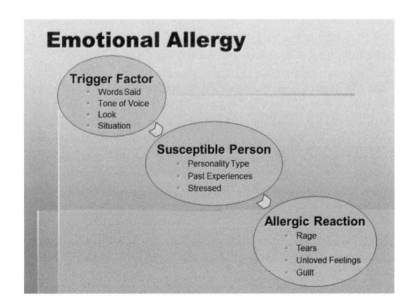

With a physical allergy, you have to figure out the cause, so you can take care of yourself. The same is true with an emotional trigger. If you don't put the time, energy and commitment into discovering what's underneath your reactions, you'll continue to experience these *emotional allergies*, or triggers, from past hurts, whether it's due to your family of origin or any long-term relationship.

Intimacy can be enhanced in any close relationship if you and your partner are guided in a process that helps you each identify your triggers, thus enabling you both to seek and offer forgiveness.

You might want to reflect on what your allergy could be. Everybody has one!

What is the root cause of emotional allergies?

It's helpful to look at them in terms of a soul wound. As an adult, you filter information. You may tell yourself, *that's garbage* or *I don't believe that*. But when you were a child, you accepted everything uncritically, and that information becomes stored in your *old brain*.

The old brain is often forgotten. You may not be aware of it until a situation arises, and you respond with a knee-jerk reaction. It brings up past hurts and is based on not having your needs met.

For me, it's when I feel not listened to or advocated for. Being aware of this emotional allergy, I self-soothe by telling myself what I'd longed to hear in my past. It helps me when that allergy strikes, and I'm overwhelmed by previous emotions. It can still hit, but instead of it having the power of Niagara Falls, it just seems like a little trickle. As some wise person once said, "You can't fix what you don't name". So, identifying it, acknowledging it and being self-compassionate through it, will help in the healing process.

You may understand by now that no one can hurt you as deeply as your loved ones. If it's an acquaintance, you can write it off, but with someone you care about, the words often stick and hurt. The wonderful flipside is that no one can heal you as much as your loved ones. You can repair your relationships if you're willing and humble enough to genuinely apologise and listen. It helps enormously in accelerating the healing process in any relationship. I love the way Henri Nouwen puts it.

"When we honestly ask ourselves which persons in our lives mean the most to us, we often find that it is those who instead of giving much advice, solutions, or cures, have chosen rather to share our pain and touch our wounds with a gentle and tender hand.

The friend who can be silent with us in a moment of despair or confusion, who can stay with us in an hour of grief and bereavement, who can tolerate not-knowing, not-curing, not-healing and face with us the reality of our powerlessness, that is the friend who cares."

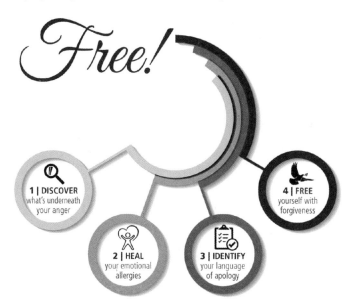

What does forgiveness mean to you?

It's interesting that the word *forgiving* can be broken up into FOR and GIVING, so you might ask, "*What* am I really giving when I forgive someone?"

The answer is that you're giving pardon to the person who wronged you. You're releasing them into the *freedom* of your forgiveness. But not only that, you're giving *yourself* freedom as well by releasing yourself from the power the hurt has over you.

The opposite of this is unresolved bitterness, which is like drinking poison and expecting the other person to die. How ridiculous is that?!

So if forgiveness is vital in maintaining a growing relationship, why is it that some apologies make the situation worse?

One of the main reasons an apology can make a situation worse is by saying "I'm sorry" without integrity.

This could happen when someone wants to get you off their back, or to make themselves feel better for having done the 'right' thing, or to move on with their life as quickly as possible.

But saying sorry for these reasons always does the relationship more harm than good in the long term.

What can stop someone from apologising?

1. **Pride**

   This is a major stumbling block to admitting wrongdoing. It takes humility to acknowledge and admit you're in the wrong.

2. **Appearing right**

   Some would rather appear right than resolve the conflict and repair the relationship.

3. **Shame**

   Many people carry huge shame, and to avoid facing it, they blame and scapegoat others.

 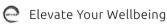

Within your counselling room, what have you found is the biggest stumbling block to apologising?

It would have to be a low self-worth, interplaying with an unconsciously held desire of having to always be right. Some people were raised in a family where the parents were always right, or they had to be perfect.

Even though your parents did the best they could with the resources they had at the time, you may have been criticised and condemned as a child, and if this issue hasn't been worked through, you might still be living with a load of shame. Sometimes hidden internal shame can be so great that you end up always having to be right. Therefore, it's really difficult to say, "I'm sorry", even with your loved ones, as it's an admission you were in the wrong.

You may have a faulty belief system that says being wrong means "I'm a failure" or "I'm inadequate" or "I'm weak." A more valid and helpful belief system is: "Being wrong means I'm human!"

When you've wronged someone in a major way, if deep repentance hasn't occurred and forgiveness isn't given, the pain resurfaces in the relationship in different ways. The feelings are still there, because they've been buried alive. It can come out as sarcasm, which is suppressed anger, or revisiting the situation. You might say, "Why are you bringing it up again? I said I was sorry".

Have you ever heard kids say "sor-RY"? This can be a sarcastic attempt at apologising without acknowledging what they're sorry for.

What are the ramifications? More salt on the wound, more brokenness to repair and more still to forgive.

When was a time you received a most heartfelt apology?

One morning, when my daughter Melinda was eight years old, she came into our bedroom, sobbing, to tell us she'd eaten the remainder of a large box of chocolates that had been left out after a Saturday night dinner party. Desperate to get it off her chest, she woke us up to convey her deep regret.

She'd consumed the chocolates and felt remorseful in less than an hour!

The problem is that adults have developed more protective layers, consisting of pride and stubbornness, that prevents them from being humble enough to admit they're in the wrong.

It's a sad state of affairs when you feel the need to hide your shame or value having to be *right* more than the relationship itself. I can still remember the look on Melinda's face. Yes, she felt great shame, but she trusted us and valued the relationship so much, she just knew there was no other option than to be honest.

What's the biggest tip you could give someone who genuinely and deeply wants to apologise to restore a relationship?

Perhaps taking the time to identify your loved one's apology language, while discovering yours as well. I could best describe it with a story about my trip to India.

My husband, John, and I were at the Taj Mahal. There were massive crowds around us, all speaking different dialects. The noise seemed like background static, or babble, until someone with an Aussie accent called out across the crowd, "Hey, Bruce". We looked up and tuned in immediately, totally focussed on his voice, because not only was someone speaking in English with an Aussie accent, but his name was Bruce!

Everybody has a primary language they use to give and receive apologies. If somebody speaks in your apology language, you will be more attuned and have a greater capacity to lean in towards the person who has wronged you.

Some people are monolingual. Others speak in all five languages but still tend to focus predominately on one or two. You might be familiar with the concept of the *Languages of Love*, which is a way of realising that people give and receive love in different ways.

You can give and receive apologies in different ways, too. Gary Chapman, in his book with Jennifer Thomas, *The Five Languages of Apology*, discusses how apologies may seem like babble to the person you've wronged. Your challenge is to make your sincere apology in the language that will seem sincere to the offended person.

What are the five languages of apology?

▶ **Language 1: Expressing Regret**

For some, receiving a sincere expression of regret is the strongest language you can use. What you don't acknowledge, you can't fix. You admit an offence has occurred, while also expressing regret for having caused the hurt, damage or injustice, when you say, "I'm really sorry for the hurt I've caused."

Some people try to skirt by with a pseudo apology that sounds like they're acknowledging the offence, but they're not. For instance, "I'm sorry you felt hurt by what happened." This kind of 'apology' has tones of denial and blame. It's not taking ownership of the offence and therefore isn't received as genuine regret.

So, expressing remorse involves more than just saying, "I'm sorry". The words need to be congruent with your body language and voice tone. The apology also needs to be specific without any 'buts'. If you offer regret then qualify it, you're shifting from an apology to an attack. Even if you have a valid point, the time to raise it is not in the midst of an apology, because it will be perceived as letting yourself off the hook.

Lesson: the language of expressing regret can't include making excuses for your offence.

▶ **Language 2: Accepting Responsibility**

I believe that any genuine apology requires a willingness to admit wrongdoing, which is an acceptance of responsibility for your actions.

For some, hearing the words "I was wrong" communicates to them that the person is sincere. One of my clients put it succinctly: "I don't need to hear 'Sorry'. I need the person to understand that *what they did was really wrong.*"

Lesson: accept full responsibility by admitting you're wrong. Don't blame anyone else or make excuses.

▶ **Language 3: Providing a Remedy**

When you've been rejected, betrayed or deeply let down, it's understandable that you need the offender to repair the damage in some way.

The words 'I'm sorry' and 'I was wrong' may not be enough. Particularly in a loving relationship, you may feel the need for your partner to make it up to you in some profound and meaningful way.

Everyone knows that actions speak louder than words, so a good apology includes a statement of willingness to remedy the situation and following through with it.

A practical example is when our daughter borrowed the car and parked it under a light pole, where a bunch of pelicans left their 'deposit' on it, thus turning our once green car white. While an apology and a promise she wouldn't do it again was nice, what we really needed was for her to wash the car! That's when we felt her genuine apology.

> ### Language 4: Being Repentant

An apology does *not* obliterate a wrong. You can't undo the past, which is why it's so important to apologise. However, you can help repair the harm you caused, so a meaningful apology needs to include an action statement as a guarantee you'll do everything in your power not to repeat the behaviour. I really value it when my husband says, "I'm going to take some action steps to try not to do this again." His intent to change, and his willingness to discuss it, just softens me.

One example of this was on a recent trip to Europe, where the amount of passive cigarette smoke was playing havoc with my lungs. I realised I couldn't request that so many people not smoke near me, especially since we were in a group, so I asked John to step in on my behalf, but he was initially reluctant. This saddened me, and I became angry. But after talking it through, and John witnessing how I was coughing and wheezing, he apologised for not taking my concerns more seriously. The following day he advocated for me, even though it made him feel awkward. Boy, did that make me feel loved! My lungs were grateful too!

> ### Language 5: Requesting Forgiveness

When forgiveness is humbly requested, it communicates that you want to repair the relationship, while also indicating you realise you did something wrong and are willing to take responsibility for it.

You can't force forgiveness. It needs to be requested, not demanded. Forgiveness is a gift, a choice to lift the penalty. It's a huge request that can be costly to the person you've hurt. In order for the relationship to be fully restored, the offended person needs to relinquish deep disappointment, and perhaps rejection, frustration, anger, embarrassment and sometimes feelings of betrayal.

They also may have to live with the consequences, such as financial issues or public humiliation. I'm conscious of how difficult it can be for a broken person to be at the same time *whole enough* to forgive. Understandably, it takes time and is a process. It's good to be mindful of this when asking someone to consider forgiving you.

Next time you make an apology, you might want to try to communicate the 5 R's.

❖ Regret

❖ Responsibility

❖ Remedy (making restitution)

❖ Repentance

❖ Request forgiveness

As Murphy's law would have it, seventy-five percent of couples differ in their apology language.

Are the 5 R's applicable only to significant relationships, or can they be applied randomly to anyone?

Any relationship, no matter what level of connection, can benefit from humble and genuine apologies. I remember when I apologised to an acquaintance I thought I'd hurt with some untimely humour. Although he said he hadn't felt offended by my words, he acknowledged how much he appreciated me caring enough to apologise anyway, and I noticed our relationship strengthened after that interaction.

I'm also reminded of a profound experience I had with a total stranger.

One time when I was cycling with a friend, I was almost wiped off my bike by a truck that swerved towards me, even though there was plenty of room to pass. When we approached the driver, he was abusive, shouting and justifying his actions by saying that it was our problem for riding on the road. After taking his registration, I reported the incident to the police, so the next innocent cyclist wouldn't be killed.

The initial response made the situation even worse. The Senior Constable was an ex truck driver and took the truckie's side. He made it clear I had no right to be on the road, and I deserved what happened to me. He did however, offer to speak to the driver, and three days later I got an amazing call from him.

Apparently the truckie had refused to come to the police station and told the officer, graphically, what he thought of him. The policeman acknowledged to me that he was wrong, said he was sorry, wanted to make up for it by writing the report and was willing to receive feedback on how he could approach these situations better in the future. He'd basically utilised all of the apology languages. Though he hadn't asked for forgiveness directly, it was implied in his actions.

I was so grateful to this random stranger demonstrating his fantastic apology skills. Think of how satisfying it would be to a loved one if you showed the same degree of care with your apology.

Are there any occasions in relationships where forgiveness is not appropriate?

Yes. In relationships where there's ongoing domestic abuse. Besides being unhelpfully premature, the strategies could be misused to reinforce the already dysfunctional positions each person holds in a relationship that's based on power and control. Understanding the domestic violence cycle is paramount here, where the perpetrator needs to take responsibility for their abusive attitudes, words and behaviours, and receive ongoing therapy and accountability to make a change. At the same time, those who've been violated need to have clear, safe and assertive choices and boundaries before any process of forgiveness can occur.

What are the stumbling blocks to forgiving?

Having attitudes of:

- I don't FEEL like it.

- They don't DESERVE it.

- I just might want to get REVENGE!

It's sad that many people don't realise how bitterness and resentment can kill the soul. Holding on to such feelings does far more damage to your own wellbeing than to the other person.

What are some of the biggest myths or misconceptions regarding forgiveness?

Forgiveness is complex and often misunderstood. These are some common misconceptions:

▸ **Forgiving means forgetting**

Why would you suddenly get amnesia, just because you've forgiven someone? In forgiving others, you're not erasing or forgetting the past but *moving on from it*. If people forgot the Holocaust, where would we be?

It's helpful to use the past memory as a *milestone* rather than a *tombstone*. A reminder of how far you've come with healing, rather than focussing on the hurt.

▸ **Forgiving condones the action**

It doesn't. It involves *letting go* of it.

▸ **Forgiveness is an emotion**

Many people believe this, and so they end up waiting years, or even a lifetime, until they *feel* like forgiving. But that day may never come. The act of forgiveness is an unnatural decision, and it's not fair. It's a challenging choice that requires grace.

Forgiveness can be a costly and complicated decision. Everyone has different leanings along the spectrum between justice and mercy. For some who hold justice highly, it can be even more difficult to choose forgiveness as an act of the will.

Walt Wangerin speaks of forgiveness as being a sort of divine absurdity. It's irrational, since the world leans toward reason.

When my clients can't seem to forgive, many of them have found it helpful to itemise the various hurts and begin by forgiving the easiest one.

When I have a hard time forgiving, I'm reminded of my faith in God, knowing all that He's gone through, in forgiving me. I reflect on His incredibly generous spirit towards me, and that really helps me get things into perspective in moving towards forgiving others.

Forgiveness *isn't:*

▸ Forgiving and forgetting

▸ A quick fix

▸ An automatic reconciliation

▸ A guarantee of change in the wrongdoer

▸ Dependent on just punishment

▸ Excusing the wrongdoer

How does forgiveness provide freedom?

By forgiving, you disinfect the wound, so the impurities have a chance to be removed, and you're able to heal.

But forgiveness takes time. It's a process that begins with an act of the will. It's not a onetime event. It's a daily choice that requires discipline and intentionality. The journey may seem to take years, but once you've released the inner pain, you can move on towards a different pathway through the freedom that forgiveness brings.

What might that freedom look or feel like?

It first involves facing your fears and accepting the challenge of refraining from a natural feeling or reaction of revenge. The actual decision to forgive can be a gut-wrenching one, but it can also feel like a supernatural process that leads to the removal of the negative feelings and thoughts towards the offender. Yes, there are painful reminders, but the freedom that forgiveness brings will enable you to remove the poison. In time, you'll notice your wounds gradually turn into scars. Just like after an operation, that scar can still give a sudden, sharp jab even years later. But in time, and with grace, you can turn those scars into stories of inspiration and encouragement for others. So not only has your own wellbeing been elevated, but you have a beautiful opportunity to be an instrument in another's wellbeing.

What is your biggest life lesson?

For me, it would have to be listening to my soul, which is my mind and emotions. I learnt a long time ago, through my psychology degree, just how powerful my thought processes are in determining my actions and the way in which I live. Yet it was only eight years ago that I personally realised the incredible significance of being in tune with my soul and giving it credibility.

In 2009 I was diagnosed with breast cancer, and for most of 2010 I was receiving heavy doses of chemotherapy and radiation after two operations to eliminate the disease. Then in 2011, when all was well with my body, I woke up from a deep sleep one night, holding both my hands on my ovaries. I sensed a voice saying, "Get your ovaries out now, Heather. Get them out NOW."

I can only describe that voice as God, but I acknowledge that many may call it their intuition.

After getting an ultrasound on my ovaries, I found out I had a precancerous tumour that made my right ovary forty-five times the size of my left one. I had them both removed immediately. Believing that God created my innermost being, I've learnt to pay close attention to His guidance. Your soul may be prompting you to apologise or even nagging you to forgive. Are you listening to those promptings?

Can you go into more detail about your freedom logo?

These are just pointers that help guide my participants in another program I've designed called *Creating Great Relationships*.

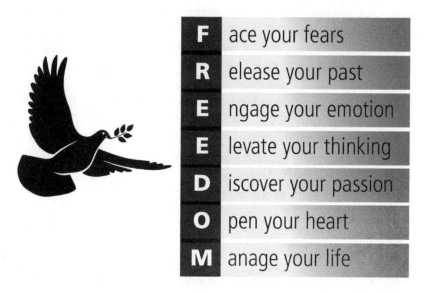

F	ace your fears
R	elease your past
E	ngage your emotion
E	levate your thinking
D	iscover your passion
O	pen your heart
M	anage your life

In particular, the first pointer, *Face your fears*, is so important in terms of forgiveness. I've heard it said that "To live with fear is a life half lived", but I don't think anyone can say it better than Nelson Mandela. Here are two quotes that were part of his 1994 Inaugural speech,

"Forgiveness liberates the soul. It removes all fear. That is why it's such a powerful weapon".

And...

"As we are liberated from our own fear, our presence automatically liberates others".

Personal growth never happens in isolation. There's always a flow-on effect. We are all people of influence. Your family relationships are instruments of influence that not only have great potential to elevate your wellbeing, but the wellbeing of those you hold dear. There are countless treasures you can leave as a legacy for your loved ones and community. Freedom through forgiveness is one of the most precious treasures you can give yourself.

 To discover more about how *Heather* can help you *Elevate Your Wellbeing,* simply visit www.elevatebooks.com/wellbeing

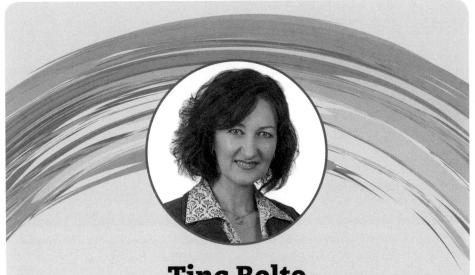

Tina Bolto

Easy Growing

Tina Bolto is the founder of Easy Growing and is a passionate food gardener and educator.

Her love of food gardening started in 1992 while assisting the establishment of a community garden. Since then, she's studied and practised various methods of growing, including organic, bio-dynamic, Permaculture and aquaponics.

She's also been a paramedic and was awarded the Australian National Medal for Service in 2013.

Tina has built two homes, one of which is a solar-passive strawbale house that was featured in Owner Builder magazine.

Having moved over thirty times, Tina is an expert in designing the perfect garden for any living situation. She's made it her mission to help others create food gardens that suit their own unique circumstance and lifestyle.

Tina Bolto

Easy Growing

What does wellbeing mean to you?

I think wellbeing is an underlying state of wellness that includes contentment, emotional stability and physical health. It means having a well-balanced, internal baseline that protects you from being reactive to every little thing that comes your way. I don't mean never feeling sad or getting sick, but that you promptly regain your wellness.

Has growing your own food contributed to your wellbeing? And if so, how?

Yes, it certainly has. My various gardens have had a significant influence on my wellbeing. Growing my own food provides me with healthy, organic produce, as well as a lot of personal satisfaction.

I find that caring for plants and connecting with nature is grounding, and even awe-inspiring. When I'm in my garden, I contemplate life. I'm often drawn to focus on the plants, produce, insects and birdlife around me, which all serve to disconnect me from stresses. It can feel like meditation. My own mindfulness exercise is concentrating on the here and now. It gives me the opportunity to put things in perspective.

> "Gardening is cheaper than therapy, and you get tomatoes."
> ~Author unknown

 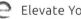

There was a time when I felt dependent and insecure, due to an abusive marriage that destroyed my self-esteem. Growing food and providing for my children gave me a huge sense of achievement, empowerment and confidence. It also provided the security of knowing we'd always have enough to eat and wouldn't have to rely on shops to keep us fed.

What is the one message you wish to share with the world?

That anyone can grow food, given the right information and resources, even if they're time poor and think they don't have a green thumb or a place to have a backyard veggie patch.

Research shows that connection with nature benefits both physical and mental health. Add to this the nutritional benefits and peace of mind of having a fresh, clean supply of produce from your own garden, and you have a strong basis for wellbeing.

Not so long ago, people grew fresh produce in home gardens; but times have changed. Nowadays, they don't have the room for fruit trees and large vegetable gardens, or the time to tend to them.

What you may not realise is that gardening is no longer as labour-intensive. New systems have been developed that simplify the process. With the right information and resources, almost anyone can reap the benefits of growing food at home, easily and efficiently.

How did you become interested in alternative gardening methods?

Through friends, teachers and moving house (a lot). And also because I don't have a green thumb.

When I moved into my first home, I planted a vegetable garden. It was down in the back corner and would get neglected whenever I was too busy or the weather was bad. Often the weeds and insect pests would get out of control, and sometimes it didn't get watered when it should have. Needless to say, it felt like too much effort at times, and it wasn't a great success. Still, picking what produce was left, felt satisfying. Peas and corn tasted sweeter, and the tomatoes were out-of-this-world delicious. So I persevered on and off for a few years with varying results, depending on the effort I could put into it.

Then I left my home, job, friends and family, and moved to the country with my two young children to escape my abusive marriage. Emotionally fragile and struggling financially, I was introduced to *Permaculture* by a friend. This changed how I looked at many aspects of daily life, and in particular to gardening.

According to Bill Mollison, who first coined the phrase, Permaculture is "the conscious design and maintenance of agriculturally productive systems, which have the diversity, stability, and resilience of natural ecosystems."

The more I learned about it, the more it encouraged me to rethink what a veggie garden looks like and ways to work with nature instead of battling against it.

About a year later, while attending a Permaculture design course, I met David Holmgren, co-originator of the Permaculture concept. When he told me this method supported rather than dictated his lifestyle choices, it influenced and inspired me. I started to consider how the various parts of my life could interact and better complement each other.

A few years after becoming qualified to teach Permaculture design, I owner-built my own home and developed an easy-care, productive food garden. The soil was poor, and I was too impatient to improve it gradually. This resulted in learning about, and experimenting with, several other methods of gardening, including raised gardens (grown in raised garden beds), wicking beds (self-contained raised beds with built-in reservoirs that supply water from the bottom up), and no-dig gardens (garden beds that are built up with layers, but not dug up or forked over).

A few years and another few moves later, I was in a small rented place and decided I didn't want to wait to own a home again before having another veggie garden. Because I worked such long hours, I was time poor, and I also didn't want to create a garden, only to leave it behind yet again.

I experimented with methods of removable gardening, including container growing and hydroponics, or growing plants without soil. This brought me to then study aquaponics, a system that combines aquaculture, which is rearing fish or other water animals, with hydroponics. In other words, the fish produce waste that feeds plants, which in turn purify the water that is then returned nice and clean to the fish. This almost-complete eco system can be largely automated and even saves water.

It was during this time that I started to plant my transportable orchard.

Moving so frequently has made me adaptable. I've been fortunate to be able to experiment with and discover the advantages and limitations of many growing methods and systems. To this day, I still apply Permaculture principles in many areas of my life, as well as using them in combination with various growing systems, to help others create their own food gardens.

What I've discovered is that there isn't one specific gardening method or system that works easily everywhere or for everyone. The best solutions must take into account environmental and lifestyle factors, as well as personal preferences. This means the best results often come from combining various methods and systems to create individualised solutions.

What is your big WHY?

When I talk to people about growing food, many say they would like to plant a garden 'one day'. This is usually followed by reasons why the time or place isn't right. For example, they're too busy and don't have room for a garden. Furthermore, as population density increases, housing affordability is reduced and the cost of living goes up, so renting is the only option for many people.

At the same time, people complain about the high cost of organic produce. But even if they are able to afford these high prices, the freshness and quality can still be significantly reduced if it's not grown locally.

I've felt those same frustrations and have discovered ways to overcome them, so now I want to inspire others to as well. I'm passionate about empowering people to improve their own health and wellbeing by providing them with the knowledge and tools to easily grow their own fresh, clean, delicious food.

You mentioned how your gardens have contributed to your emotional wellbeing. What other benefits are there to growing your own food?

The most obvious benefit of home-grown food is freshness. You can see, feel and taste the difference. Just-picked, home-grown fruit and vegetables will always be much fresher than commercial produce. Freshness affects the nutrient content of food, as well as the taste and other qualities.

Commercial produce must be harvested, processed (washed and/or waxed), packaged, stored and transported, often over large distances, even to other countries. Then there's shop shelf time, followed by home storage prior to preparation and consumption.

Some 'fresh' produce can take months before it gets to your local shop. Apples, for example, can be harvested and then kept in cold storage for up to a year before being available for sale in the supermarket! The following list shows some of the produce that can be stored before being sold as fresh many weeks later.

Produce Item	Acceptable commercial storage period
Grapes	26 weeks
Apples	52 weeks
Lemons	26 weeks
Pears	30 weeks
Pumpkin	18 weeks
Cabbage	4 weeks
Chinese cabbage	12 weeks
Carrots	26 weeks
Celeriac	40 weeks
Garlic	30 weeks
Ginger	26 weeks
Leeks	8 weeks
Lettuce, iceberg	4 weeks
Lettuce, loose leaf	2 weeks
Parsley	8 weeks
Parsnip	26 weeks
Potato	26 weeks
Snow peas	3 weeks
Turnip (& Swedes)	20 weeks

So how do they keep apples crisp for up to a year after harvest?

It's because they're harvested before they ripen and then kept cold in a controlled atmosphere (CA). They're also (generally) treated with 1-methylcyclopropene (1-MCP, often called SmartFresh) to prevent them from ripening by blocking the ethylene receptors.

Produce can also be treated to prevent fungal rot. Although Smartfresh isn't approved for use on organic produce, some fungicides are. Even organic apples may be kept in cold storage to extend availability beyond the usual seasons.

While these treatments can be effective, there's a significant loss of quality and nutritional value during storage. Vitamin C breaks down rapidly from the time fruit and vegetables are harvested, and it continues to decline while in storage. Because vitamin C content is easily measured, it's often used as a way of calculating nutritional changes in fruit and vegetables. B-vitamins, including thiamine and vitamin B-6, are particularly sensitive to nutritional decline during transport and storage.

Polyphenols are antioxidants found in high levels in fresh apples, pears, peaches and blueberries. They've been shown to lower cholesterol and blood pressure, improve arterial function, help fight cancer and increase life span. But polyphenol content progressively decreases during prolonged storage times, including cold storage.

Because produce loses its nutritional value following harvest, fruit and vegetables purchased from retailers will have lost many more nutrients than home-grown, freshly picked produce.

There's also evidence that machine harvesting causes more shock to the plants than hand harvesting, which means increased metabolism that leads to a quicker loss of nutrients and deterioration of quality.

In addition to nutritional benefits, fresh home-grown produce is often superior in taste and texture. Fresh-picked peas, for example, taste sweeter than those purchased in shops. This is due to an increase in starch after they're picked. There are several other reasons home-grown produce is superior, most of them based on the needs of commercial production and financial profits.

1-MCP treatment, which again is used to extend storage and shelf life, has been found to reduce flavour and aroma development when the fruit eventually ripens.

Varieties of produce grown by commercial producers are selected for different qualities than those likely to be chosen by home gardeners. The following table outlines some of the commercial preferences and reasons for them, compared to the benefits of home gardening.

Commercial Preference	Reason for Commercial Preference	Home Gardening Preference	Home Gardening Benefits
Fruit all matures together over a short period	Harvesting can be done *en-masse* for labour and time efficiencies. (In addition, it can then be kept in a controlled atmosphere to extend availability to consumers.)	Gradual ripening to allow genuinely fresh produce to be harvested regularly throughout the season.	Harvesting time can be further extended by planting over a longer period, such as a few more lettuce heads every couple of weeks, or by planting varieties that fruit at different times. For instance, Navel oranges for winter and Valencia oranges for summer.

Commercial Preference	Reason for Commercial Preference	Home Gardening Preference	Home Gardening Benefits
Strong skin and/or firm flesh	Tougher produce resists damage from processing and handling and is delivered undamaged to retail stores.	Taste, texture and variety can be chosen over the need to meet commercial production requirements.	Many varieties of fruits and vegetables have superior taste and other qualities. Also, many soft skin fruits aren't readily available commercially, such as loquats, *feijoas*, cumquats and persimmons.
Uniformity of appearance	Consumer preference for uniform, aesthetically pleasing produce.	Selecting alternative varieties adds interest, as well as taste.	Can grow over 3,000 heirloom varieties of tomatoes, as well as purple carrots or beans, dozens of pumpkin varieties and miniature vegetables.
Disease and pest resilience	Monoculture and intensive farming practices encourage attacks from pests and disease. Damaged produce reduces profitability.	Less intensive growing and crop rotation significantly reduces the damage done by pests and disease. Home gardeners may also accept slight imperfections, like spots on apples, in order to reduce or eliminate chemical contamination.	Other ways to reduce pests and disease in the home garden without the use of chemicals include companion planting, encouraging beneficial insects and providing alternative food sources. For instance, snails and slugs are attracted to beer and then drown.

Try the tomato drop test. Take a commercial vine- ripened truss tomato in one hand and a ripe home-grown heirloom (old traditional variety) tomato in the other. Hold them both at head height and drop them onto a hard surface. The commercial tomato is likely to bounce or roll, with its skin remaining intact. The heirloom tomato has probably split open or squashed, spilling out its juicy contents.

So what does this mean to the home gardener? Taste tests tell! Numerous comparisons continue to prove that heirloom varieties of tomatoes have far superior taste and texture to commercial varieties.

Many people also grow their own food to protect themselves and their families from exposure to, and ingestion of, chemicals and poisons. Generally, commercial produce must rely on the use of chemical pesticides, herbicides, fungicides and fertilisers during production, to maximize yield and profits. Some crops have even been bred to tolerate exposure to high concentrations of chemicals. For example, Round-up Ready seeds developed by Monsanto allow high concentrations of glyphosate herbicide to be used without damaging the commercial crop.

Reducing exposure and eliminating ingestion of these chemicals is the primary aim of choosing organic (or biodynamic) over conventional food and products. But purchasing organic produce can be costly. The growers rely on methods of agriculture and management that are more labour intensive and can also result in reduced yields when compared to conventional methods.

By growing your own food organically, with the assistance of natural methods of pest control, it's possible to reduce or eliminate ingestion of chemical contaminants. The decreased need to purchase commercial organic produce can also save you money.

There are many more reasons you might choose to grow your own food. Some are universal, some are of personal importance, while others could be environmental. Here are some common motivations:

1. Convenience

Not having to go out to the shops and being able to pick and eat from your own garden. This is especially fun for children.

2. Education

Witnessing the miracle of life through planting a tiny seed, caring for it and watching it transform into a plant, ready to be picked and eaten.

Children can observe how peas grow and dig for potatoes hidden under the ground. If you've only grown up on store-bought peas, you may not even be aware they grow in pods on vines. There are lots of fun lessons to learn in a food garden.

3. Choice

You have access to fruit and vegetable varieties that have the qualities you want most, rather than those that suit commercial needs. There are several companies that supply a wide variety of seeds by mail.

4. Reduced fossil fuel consumption

Transport distances are a major consideration in calculating the indirect costs to the environment and depletion of non-renewable resources.

5. Reduced soil degradation

Using sustainable agricultural practices in the home garden can reduce or eliminate erosion and loss of topsoil. Intensive commercial agriculture may also cause depletion of minerals and trace elements in soil.

There are other indirect personal benefits to gardening. You might love to share your produce with family and friends and feel good about providing healthy, clean, nutritious food to your loved ones.

There can also be a sense of pride in the achievement of creating a garden that's unique and/or innovative, as well as the pleasure of successfully growing your own food.

Or you may strive for self-sufficiency and having the freedom and security of no longer relying on commercial production.

So why don't more people have vegetable gardens?

After asking many people this question, I've discovered that most of it comes back to lifestyle changes.

The convenience of supermarkets, grocery stores and mass commercial food production means that food is available without the need for a garden. But this is at a cost, which is compromised food quality for commercial profit.

So overall, many people believe they don't have the time or space for a food garden, or that it will take too much effort. But what they don't realise is that it's now easier than ever to grow their own food.

Does a home garden need to be organic?

My personal preference is to grow food organically.

However, I understand organic gardening isn't for everyone, so if you decide to use chemicals in your home garden, it's important to avoid exposure and/or consumption of toxic substances on your produce. Here are some guidelines to help minimize your risk.

- Always follow the manufacturer's directions.

- Observe safety recommendations, including wearing a mask, eye protection and gloves.

- Don't be tempted to use stronger concentrations above the recommended dilutions.

- Be sure to observe withholding times. That is, produce sprayed with some chemicals can't be consumed for a particular period from the time the chemical was used.

- Always wash your produce prior to consumption, preparation or storage. I recommend using water with a dash of dish washing liquid, as this helps to remove oily residues. Then rinse this off as well.

What's the biggest mistake people make when they decide to grow vegetables at home?

I notice that a lot of the struggling veggie gardens are put in a corner down at the bottom of the backyard. That's what I did at first as well

There are a few problems with this approach. In fact, this kind of garden isn't ideal for most people. The back corner might not be optimal for plant growth and is probably not the most convenient location for easy upkeep.

As for the neat rows, I've found that combined gardens are less labour intensive and more productive, except for corn, as it needs to be closely planted in order to cross pollinate via wind. Combined gardens usually have less pest problems as well. Imagine a cabbage moth, looking for the distinct grey-green of cabbages upon which to lay her caterpillar eggs. If they're planted amongst carrots and silver beet, they will be less of a beacon.

Based on your experience, what's the biggest tip you could give to home gardeners?

Don't change your life to grow your garden; create a garden that fits into your life!

My best advice is to first consider your day-to-day activities.

How do you want to utilise your outdoor space? For instance, I entertain once a year at most, so for me a large entertaining area is a waste of space. Instead, I grow fruit trees and have social gatherings at other locations.

Do you need a lawn or fenced-in play area for the children and/or a dog? What about when you have guests over or desire a quiet place to sit and read?

Everyone has different needs for their outdoor space, which is why one size does not fit all when it comes to food gardens.

Also consider where you frequently traverse or spend time. For instance, the convenience of picking some salad greens on your way into your home after checking your letterbox. Or maybe you have a patio where you could grow herbs close to your kitchen.

Do you have an approach that can help people create a garden that works for them?

Yes. I call it my *Stop, Get ready, Grow* system. In my courses, I use a traffic light and apples to depict the steps.

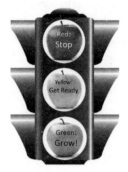

Step One: Stop (Red apple)
Evaluate your current situation (lifestyle).
- What are the advantages?
- What are the challenges?
- What are your resources?
- What are your priorities?

Step Two: Get Ready (Yellow apple)
Examine information to make educated decisions.
- Evaluation of growing systems
- Introduction to Permaculture
- Consideration of complementary systems

Step Three: Grow! (Green apple)
Make your final decision regarding your food plants.
- What to grow
- What not to grow
- How to grow

In my experience, many people head straight to the grow step, or even to the very last section on what and how to grow food, but going through the steps in order is essential.

I'd like to share with you some details from the first, and most important, step: *Stop*.

The information gathered when you stop and evaluate your current situation, resources and preferences, makes all the difference in deciding what you will grow, as well as where and how you will grow it. This avoids wasting time, energy and money later, and it's the basis for creating a garden that works for you and your unique situation.

Let's start by slicing your red *Stop* apple into quarters.

The first two slices of apple represent the **advantages and challenges** of your current living situation. This section is about you and the place you live.

I suggest spending at least ten minutes on each of these. The idea is to list as many as you can.

Below is an example of entries for Karen. She's renting and is a single mother with two young children. Here is her list of all possible advantages and challenges regarding her current situation.

Advantages	**Challenges**
I'm good at putting things together, like Ikea furniture.	I don't have a strong partner to help with heavy work.
I'm patient.	I need space for the children to play.
I have spare time while children are at school.	Financial challenges. Need to plan expenditure over time.
Children are keen to help.	Clay soil gets water logged.
Landlord will allow me to use old veggie patch down the back.	Need space for the dog.
Long-term lease. Am likely to stay here a few years.	Renting.
Landlord will allow me to use garden beds around the lawn and out the front for growing food.	Landlord will not allow me to use lawn area back and front for growing food.
Wide front veranda is sunny until late afternoon all Winter.	Backyard is mostly shaded all summer from large deciduous tree.

The third slice of the apple is for **resources.** Here are some that Karen could tap into.

- Large rainwater tank, as well as township water supply
- Helpful friends
- Manure from friend's horse
- Borrowed trailer
- Nearby garden centre
- Free pallets from local hardware store
- Tools (hammer, saw, drill)
- Garden tools (rake, small hand spade and fork). Can also borrow wheelbarrow and spade/shovel
- Local gardening group will share seeds and cuttings. (Look up groups through Meet-up, check with local council and search on Facebook)
- Pile of old bricks, timbers, posts, heavy-duty plastic and old carpet

The fourth slice is **priorities.**

This is where you consider your priorities and list them from most to least important.

The best way I've found to do this is by first brainstorming to create a list. I've provided some examples in the left column below. You can start with these and add more of your own.

Next, quickly glance through your list and pick out the one item that stirs the most emotion within you. Put this at the top of the right column. Repeat the process for choosing the next one that stands out, until the column on the right is full and contains all of your prioritised considerations.

Note: by doing this quickly, without thinking or contemplating, you're more likely to come up with the most emotionally significant, rather than rational, answers. You can review and reorder them if necessary, but be aware that your underlying emotional or subconscious preferences are more likely to reflect your deeper needs than your rational preferences.

Again, using Karen as an example:

Brain Storming List	**Prioritised List**
• Chemical-free foods	• Chemical-free foods
• Teach children about real food and nature	• Save money
• Spend time with children	• Getting children outside
• Get the children outside	• Teaching children
• Save money	• Spending time with children
• Time efficiency	• Convenience
• Convenience	• Time efficiency

Here are some examples of how the information you gather when you stop to evaluate your current situation and priorities can be used in the development of an individualised system plan:

1. A single mother with school-aged children, but limited financial resources, might decide to start small, using resources she already has access to. She could start with rapidly maturing crops like radishes, rainbow chard (coloured silver beet) and cherry tomatoes to keep the children's interest, and then later expand the garden gradually over time.

2. A busy single person renting a north-facing, upstairs flat might decide on a slim Ballerina apple and a heavy cropping miniature fruit tree, and grow them in self-watering pots. Loving homemade

pizza, they might also grow tomatoes and herbs in pots or hanging baskets. It may even be possible to grow some plants indoors.

3. An inland rural family relying on rainwater with risk of drought, might set up an aquaponics system in a greenhouse to grow all their fruit, vegetables, salad greens and even herbs, because the water is constantly being recycled with little loss or waste. The system could be automated, and as a bonus, they could also have fresh fish to eat.

4. Someone with access to manure and bedding straw from stables, might choose to entirely fill a raised bed with the mix and plant directly into it once it's composted, rather than purchasing garden soil to fill garden beds.

It sounds like there are quite a few options. How do people find a method that suits them?

By gathering and examining information, you can make an educated decision. Once you have all of your *Stop* information, you will be able to consider different methods and systems for suitability in your own circumstances.

I go into more detail about this in my workshops, but in step two, the *Get ready* (yellow apple) section, is where you decide on the planting method that works best for you, based on the information you collected in step one. For instance, you might consider the advantages and disadvantages of up to twenty different growing methods and systems, from traditional garden plots to no-dig gardens, hydroponics and aquaponics, to wicking beds and vertical gardens. Each is suited to different people and circumstances.

Then there are choices like the conventional, organic or bio-dynamic methods, not to mention companion planting, where certain plants are known to be mutually beneficial. There's also moon planting, where lunar cycles are considered in order to optimise development.

I also encourage the use of some Permaculture principles to help you consider how your garden can integrate with other aspects of your life. When you're ready, you can move forward to the *Grow* step with confidence, knowing that the method, or combination of methods, will give you the best results, which is fresh, healthy, nutritious produce that's convenient and fits into your lifestyle.

Whatever your circumstance and preferences, your perfect system will be one that's personalised to suit you, bringing you pleasure and health, and contributing to your wellbeing.

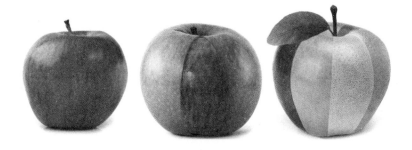

"The glory of gardening: hands in the dirt, head in the sun, heart with nature. To nurture a garden is to feed not just on the body, but the soul." ~Alfred Austin

 To discover more about how *Tina* can help you *Elevate Your Wellbeing,* simply visit www.elevatebooks.com/wellbeing

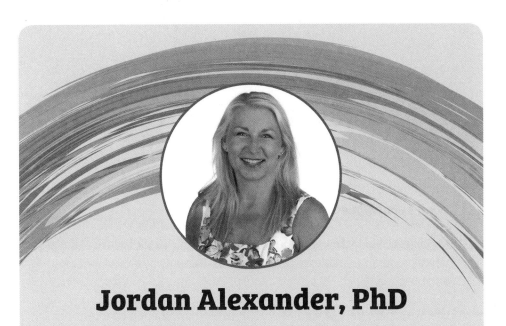

Jordan Alexander, PhD

Foundation Love

Jordan Alexander is an author, educator and facilitator who brings visions to life. As managing director at Pangaea Consulting, she's helped transform thousands of lives across government, business and community sectors. Her coaching and courses enrich and inspire.

Born in Canada to Croatian and Ukrainian immigrants, Jordan became fascinated with how culture shapes mindset and delved into the subject of unconscious bias while achieving her PhD.

Her research and experience provided the catalyst for The UBU Practice™, a simple, holistic, and effective methodology that helps people find their authentic voice, articulate their dreams and align their lifestyle. Her coaching practice, Love Assist Associates, helps relationship seekers find authentic love connections.

Jordan lives in Wellington with her husband and two daughters.

Jordan Alexander, PhD

Foundation Love

What's your biggest life lesson?

My biggest life lesson is eloquently captured by Viktor Frankl: "Life is never made unbearable by circumstances, but only by lack of meaning and purpose."

Life events are part of an elaborate master plan, shaped by intentions and unwrapped in divine synchronicity. During a marriage breakup, health scare or work restructure, it may be challenging to find meaning and purpose. Reflecting afterward, you'll find lessons or develop a better understanding of how events change your life course and realise it's the best thing that could have happened.

I know I found meaning and purpose while reflecting on a family adversity, one that shaped who I am today.

When I was twenty-one, I attended June graduation at Queen's University in Kingston, Ontario. My alcoholic father didn't make it. He was in our hometown getting another blood transfusion.

STOP wasn't a word *Tata* used when he was drinking, not even when fighting for his life. His liver, on the other hand, discovered the true meaning of it. He died with no will, no life insurance and no cash. The cemetery didn't take a credit card, so I sold my Trans Am to pay for his burial plot. After the funeral, I deferred law school to support my family as the new Marijan's Garage proprietor. At the time I thought, *How can I possibly run an auto body shop with a BA in geography?*

The circumstances seemed unbearable, but I had to find my courage and figure out a way to put food on the table. My purpose, to care for my family, made me grow stronger out of necessity. I became resourceful, recycling truck engine oil as an under-spray for cars to protect them from salt on winter roads and carrying scrap metal in our dodgy-brakes tow truck to the junkyard to get cash for groceries.

Each night I'd fall into bed exhausted, but increasingly proud of my efforts. Manual labour, much to my surprise, turned out to be satisfying. I found meaning and purpose in what initially seemed an insufferable circumstance. The impact of my dad's death was emotionally harsh, but the totality of the circumstance taught me so much about myself, people and life. I learned how to dig deep, never give up and that anything is possible.

What does love mean to you?

If I could take only one word away with me on a desert island, *love* would be it. This amazing, ubiquitous four-letter word captures everything from how I feel about pizza and chocolate, to my daughters, lover, family and friends. Experiencing love is like flying upside down in one of those old crop-dusting planes while your oxygen mask is filled with laughing gas. It's intoxicating, humbling and overwhelming at the same time; a mind-body-soul orgasm.

Love is the foundation for absolutely everything human beings are about. It constantly expands and gets deeper and stronger with age. It's why I started *Love Assist Associates*—a company dedicated to helping one million genuine love seekers find their authentic love connection by 2025.

There's an endless supply of love, like some renewing gift-with-procreation purchase. Yet access to it can be elusive. When you're trying too hard to find love, it will insist that you surrender before it will readily embrace you. I refer to this giving/receiving equation as the *yin* and *yang* of love. Self-love is an essential building block to receiving, as it connects you to your soul, thus enabling the base to let love in. Learning self-love is the key to successful relationships and sits at the heart of *Love Assist Associates* and *The UBU Practice*.

If you were speaking to your younger self, what advice would you give?

I would say...

Rather than demanding immediate answers, send your questions out to the universe and let go. Trust that the solution will find you. Forcing action, rather than waiting patiently, undermines the natural unfolding of the rhythm of life. Answers come in the quiet.

Relax into it, let go and remember...*All things in time.*

What's the one message you wish to share with the world?

Believe in yourself.

I want everyone in the world to be their authentic self and speak their truth, appreciate their limitless potential and understand that if they can dream it, they can do it. I want them to follow their heart and find the courage to live the life they've always imagined.

I believe in you. I want to hear you say with conviction, "I got this!" because you believe in yourself enough. Until then, I'll be the one in your ear whispering (in a compelling but supportive voice), "YOU GOT THIS!"

What's the worst thing that's ever happened to you, and how did you overcome it?

The worst thing that ever happened to me was spending half my life disconnected from my soul, living every, and anyone else's reality, because I lacked the self-confidence, self-respect and self-love needed to be free and be me.

During my childhood, rather than being carefree and living my own truth, I was figuring out how to survive all kinds of abuse. Growing up in an alcoholic family doesn't engender strong emotional attachments with others, including your own parents, who are part of the cycle. Couple that with experiences a young child should never be exposed to, nor endure, and you end up acquiring limiting beliefs, no sense of self-worth or respect, and a warped understanding of love and relationships. The environment wasn't a secure one, so I protected myself—my authentic me—by building a wall and crawling behind it to stay safe. My story isn't unique. Others live behind their own safety wall, cut off from living their bliss.

Here's how I overcame my *worst thing*.

Five years ago, my inauthentic life culminated while shopping in Waikiki Beach in Hawaii. I went there after the universe gave me an unexpected wakeup call in the form of a romance scam (read: *iloveyousendmoney.com*). The experience left me broken financially, spiritually and emotionally. At rock bottom, I came across the book *She* and opened it at a page that read...*She realised that she was the one she was waiting for.* Talk about a smack across the head. That's when I realised there was no knight in shining armour coming to save me from the burning turret. And even if he did exist, his quest was futile, as I was the relentless arsonist in my own life.

This spurred me on to throw away the matches, tear down the brick wall, and try to discover where I lost myself. That book was the catalyst that led me to create *The UBU Practice*, a how-to guide to blast away limiting beliefs, create a new relationship with yourself and practice living an authentic life. It worked for me, and I want to share my *Discover. Explore. Grow.* methodology with you, so you can also love living your own authentic life.

What's your big WHY?

Helping people transform, grow and achieve their dreams is my WHY. My life is dedicated to inspiring others to find their authentic self, live their authentic life and experience the ripple of their passion enriching our global community.

My experience exploring different places and working with amazing people in incredible organisations, businesses and charities, has allowed me to hone my skill at cutting through the noise to get to the core goal or dream, germinating amidst complicated ideas or messy problems. Revealing a simple and clear path for others to grow and live their passions, gives me extreme personal satisfaction and joy. I like being part of the support crew, encouraging and inspiring people to transform and live a life they don't need a vacation from.

What are you passionate about?

I'm passionate about cultures and beliefs and how they influence people. Everyone grows up in a set of *matryoshka* dolls, those Russian nesting figures that fit into each other. Your authentic self is in the middle, surrounded by family, culture, nation and geography. You develop and grow, nestled within these interconnected layers. To understand yourself, you need to discern and align your authentic beliefs.

I was born in Canada, a country with a rich multicultural mosaic, different from our adjacent American melting pot. My heritage added to the cultural mix, as my Ukrainian mother, an Orthodox believer, told the story of her marriage in 1966 to my Croatian father, a Roman Catholic. The mixing of religions influenced several close friends and family to boycott their wedding. I never understood the controversy, since both were Christians.

I enjoyed the diversity, perhaps since it meant celebrating Christmas and Easter twice. As a child, I was mesmerised by Easter Sunday mass at the Orthodox Church with my *babushka* (grandmother) carrying Easter baskets filled with *pysanky* (painted eggs), homemade *kielbasa* and *paska* (sweet bread), all wrapped in hand-embroidered, black and red cross-stitched linen. The *svyschenyk* (priest) would walk through rows of baskets, with incense wafting through the open air.

On my father's side, my Croatian relatives would tenaciously correct me when I referred to my Yugoslavian heritage (I was born during Tito's rule), but I didn't appreciate the nationality distinction until visiting Zagreb post-war in 1997.

Cultural diversity, richness and misunderstanding exist on many levels. I realised the extent of inherent cultural bias when I became involved in planning, policy and consulting roles across North America and Australasia. Because I'd been raised and educated in a Western system, until that point I'd had little exposure to other cultural philosophies.

I witnessed indigenous beliefs repeatedly disregarded and superseded by Western translations, particularly around land issues. As these conflicts continued, I felt compelled to find answers to the question of how to bridge cultural gaps and varied perceptions.

During my PhD, I delved into the worldview of different nations that influenced the American town of Sitka, Alaska, including the Native American *Tlingit* and colonial Russian history. I explored the systematised views of worldly phenomena such as love, life, death, priorities and values, which gave me fascinating insights into identity and neural wiring. My personal transformation included learning to pause and ask questions about inherent beliefs and my perception of people and places.

Opening your own *matryoshka* doll can reveal a wider context that will help you establish a deeper connection to your authentic self. Actively shedding what no longer suits or aligns with who you want to be, can direct your journey to celebrate your own diversity. You'll also develop a greater appreciation of our vibrant global society.

What do you think people's biggest life issues are?

Most major issues, whether in relationships, career, mindset or health, stem from disconnection with the authentic self and our built-in compass. When you swim upstream, away from your authentic life, passion and soul's purpose, you can get frustrated with the 'You are here' scenario and be unclear as to how you got to this dispassionate place. The Talking Heads song, 'Once in a Lifetime', captures this emotion, in which you tell yourself "This is not my beautiful house" and ask yourself, "How did I get here?" Discontent then becomes the norm, and fear kicks in to prevent change. It keeps you stuck in "same as it ever was".

Based on your experience, what's the best tip you could give?

Back yourself.

Being true to your authentic self allows you to discern and jettison parts of your disconnected life that are preventing you from living your passions and dreams. When you back yourself, you're connected and make decisions that feel right. As a result, life unfolds naturally, without resistance. Part of *The UBU Practice* is creating a *Self-Love Bubble*. It strengthens your connection with your authentic self, helping to grow your courage and confidence to support living your bliss.

What's your most inspiring client story?

My client, The Billy Graham Youth Foundation (BGYF), is my most inspiring story. I love how Billy overcame personal hardship to change the lives of young people in his community and across Aotearoa (New Zealand).

I met Billy in 2013 when *The Tindall Foundation* commissioned me to independently assess the potential to expand Billy's Naenae Boxing Academy (NBA) across the country. Billy, a former Australasian boxing champion, founded NBA in 2006 as a fitness-based development program targeting at-risk youth. Young people learn boxing skills, reach their potential and make a valuable contribution within their communities.

As a consultant, I could see the wider benefits in health outcomes through exercise and sport, and by targeting at-risk youth, it made good social investment sense as well. Prevention reduces youth justice detention and rehabilitation costs. A non-resident placement is $22,000 per person, while three months in-residence is $123,000.

Comparatively, NBA delivers at $2,000 per member. It has strong support from NZ Police and youth justice judges, and has captured international attention with successful crime prevention statistics, positive participant feedback and the dynamic presence of Billy Graham at its heart.

My challenge was to explore the feasibility of replicating Billy's magic, without having to clone him. I needed to capture his essence while developing an operating model to spread the spirit, and at the same time build strong, sustainable communities. The Feasibility Study included an implementation plan to establish 'the first three' new academies. Unlike many reports that people put on a shelf and forget, this dedicated team just got on with the mission: *Empowering youth to be the best they can be.*

How could I not stay involved?! Thousands of young people have been through the boxing gyms already. Kids from all walks of life, including those at-risk with gang or drug-related issues. They spend a few years attending the boxing academy and come out the other side talking about how it changed their lives.

In 2016, I became trustee and chair of the Billy Graham Youth Foundation. We knew the formula was working but needed evidence to prove it. We commissioned Victoria University to provide an independent evaluation, which confirmed the model works. In 2018, I stepped down after the successful installation of five gyms across the country.

The gratitude I feel by contributing even a small part to making dreams a reality, is bliss. Recalling success stories from our young people, and seeing Billy's face light up as his vision came to life, makes me smile from my heart. I will dine on this *inspiring client story* for the rest of my life.

How did you decide on the name and logo for your business?

My business equips people with the know-how to live their dream life. Essentially, getting you in touch with how...you...be...you (UBU). Your UBU transformation begins with a retreat, workshop or online program where you *Discover. Explore. Grow.* your authentic voice, articulate your goals and align your lifestyle. UBU is a *practice* as well as a program, so your journey continues through daily exercises that create deeper and stronger connections for you and your authentic life.

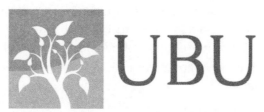

Wayne Dyer used to talk about the 'tree-ness' of the mighty oak held within the acorn. UBU supports your journey into your *tree-ness*.

The tree logo captures the unique characteristics of people. At once, a tree embraces the flexible *willow*, delicate *frangipani*, strong *kauri* and versatile *koru* (silver fern). Each is influenced by roots and experiences, grows in different ways and places, and is born to fulfil a unique destiny.

How would you describe the approach for your personal transformation program?

The UBU Practice involves three steps that build on my *Beliefs Model,* including invisible elements like neural programming, behaviour changes and more tangible information gathered through the senses. Here's an overview:

▶ **Step 1: Get naked to expose your authentic roots**

Your authentic roots contain your cultural heritage and lived experiences. The influences that have shaped your 'You are here.' To help you get naked with your authentic self, we apply the *Discover. Explore. Grow.* methodology to jettison excess baggage and self-limiting beliefs. You clarify your authentic values and use these signposts for lifestyle choices and throughout your transformation journey.

▶ **Step 2: Design your Self-Love Bubble to fortify your base**

Your base (tree trunk) is decision-making central, containing your head, heart and gut/instinct. You filter what comes through your roots by designing your unique Self-Love Bubble with brain rewiring, gut soulfulness and heart balancing.

For instance, if you've been making decisions in life based on your head, you've probably built an impermeable wall of protection around your heart. This makes it difficult to digest anything going on in your life, such as abuse, emotions, attachment or authenticity, so your emotional guidance system is in need of a clean-out.

Keeping your connection to self—that link between your soul's bliss and day-to-day practical realities—is aided by your Self-Love Bubble daily rituals, like yoga and meditation. The Bubble gives you permission to allow your heart to sing with joy and love. In your Bubble, someone always has their pompoms out cheering for you, supporting you, keeping your winning mindset at the fore. It acts like Gandalf, protecting you with the warning, "Self-limiting beliefs shall not pass..."

Designing your own Self-Love Bubble will fortify your base and allow you to venture out, develop healthy emotional connections and learn to trust your intuition.

▶ ### Step 3: Branch out to make a difference living your dream

A branch is where your authentic self reaches out and touches the world. It's shaped by your *tree-ness* and the place you identify as home. There are five UBU branches:

1. **Your Calling**

   • Applying your unique talents to a career/vocation.

2. **A Positive Attitude**

   • Living with fun, gratitude and happiness.

3. **Love & Relationships**

   • Genuine, meaningful connections with others.

4. **Mindful Self-Connection**

   • Being supported by your Self-Love Bubble.

5. **Health & Wellness**

   • Physical strength and agility, good nutrition and movement.

 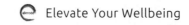

How and when you develop your branches depends on your journeying. One of my favourite watercolours of Old Quebec features the seasonal transformation of a birch tree. It serves as a reminder of cyclical change, different life stages, events and experiences. Applying the *Discover. Explore. Grow.* methodology raises awareness around lifestyle choices to align your transformation and authentic UBU journey.

My calling is to assist people in discovering their *tree-ness*, getting naked with their authentic roots and connecting their authentic self to their unique journey. The best way I know to achieve this is by supporting personal transformations using *The UBU Practice*.

What courses/training have you done that enabled you to get started or build your business?

I'm a one-hundred-percent committed lifelong learner, utilising a combination of academic research and practical learning opportunities. I've had formal university training in Canada and New Zealand to a doctorate level, which enabled a strong theoretical underpinning for the UBU curriculum. I supplement higher education with practical business experience. Clients and colleagues constantly stretch my thinking and allow me to test and combine theory and practice.

I've taken many courses through Authentic Education. Learning by doing, is so important in our fast-paced world. Ben and Cham offer great content and solid support pre and post-workshops.

Lastly, nothing provides better training than walking through the fire. It wasn't always easy. To align my life and lifestyle with my passion, I had to go through an identity crisis and lose my heart a few times...as well as my head...along with lots of money. But I wouldn't change a thing. I needed to learn how to swallow hard, be brave, cry and release. You can't learn perseverance in a book! If I hadn't gone through all of that and lived to tell the story, what lessons would I have to share to help others?!

Do you live your love?

Absolutely. I'm blessed and grateful for my life and the people in it.

Sometimes I feel like a fairy godmother, granting wishes. My life is about making people's dreams come true. Each year just keeps taking me to higher realms of satisfaction and happiness, personally and professionally.

I stepped back from a lucrative management consulting career to refocus on individuals, which meant moving from helping organisations align their people, to helping individuals align who they are. In some ways, it's same-same; in others, it's totally different. Rather than shoehorn people into someone else's dream, I'm helping them discover and grow their own. This doesn't mean that people's dreams can't align with organisations. What it does mean is that people need a more active and deliberate alignment to their authentic self.

The marriage of passion and career is a beautiful union. I love helping others create this connection. I believe this is my purpose.

How can people be happier in life?

Always do your best.

When I was a little girl in Guiding, I promised to *do my best, to do my duty to God, the Queen and my country, and to help other people every day, especially those at home*. I didn't know it then, but the *always do your best* mindset is a direct route to happy. When you give it your all and know you couldn't have tried any harder, you will always be proud of your effort, irrespective of the outcome. And for those days when you think of settling for mediocrity...dig deep, and leave it all on the track. You'll be glad you did and be infinitely happier in life.

What are your favourite ways to relax and enjoy your life?

Relaxing and getting energised at the same time sounds like a contradiction, but my favourite ways to unwind act like power naps for my soul's joy.

The extroverted me loves being with people. I wholeheartedly embrace the Maori proverb, *"He tangata! He tangata! He tangata!"* Translation: It's people! It's people! It's people! Experiencing diverse cultures while sharing food, wine, love, and especially laughter, calms me as I sink into different worlds, lives and perceptions. Engaging with people energises me and emphasises the invisible thread that connects us. I revel in how anything is possible...together.

The introverted me loves taking time out on or near water, communing with nature and being outdoors. In windy Wellington, unless there's a typhoon, I'm outside gazing at my harbour for inspiration. Books, music and art are my chill-out desserts, and stillness, my palate cleanser.

Slowing down strengthens my self-love connection, clarifies my soul's purpose and energizes me to go forth, make a difference and enjoy living.

What tools would you recommend to people struggling to stay focused, especially if progress is slow or barriers threaten their goals and dreams?

Two things will keep you focused: faith and connection to self.

There's a quote I love by Elisabeth Eliot: "Don't dig up in doubt what you planted in faith." What this means is that faith will keep you focused with unfaltering belief in the future, and you need to trust in order to know that the universe's *apparent* roadblock has appeared to help you collect an essential piece for your future picture.

Self-care resides in your Self-Love Bubble, which is especially important during busy or trying times, like when you're realigning your life.

I tell all my clients, "You can have the most elegant strategy, but success or failure always comes down to implementation." Goals are important, as they point you in the direction of where you want to be, but without enabling an implementation strategy, you'll always fall short of achieving your full potential.

What's one strategy someone could use right now to change their life?

Forgive yourself and others.

There's a frailty to being human that begs for compassion and empathy when you stuff things up, make poor choices or have bad hair days. Everyone needs forgiveness.

Holding a grudge (being unforgiving) is the biggest barrier to success, keeping you stuck by clogging your heart and mind. Forgiving releases expectations that the past will repeat itself. I wasted thirty years angry with my mom for not providing a Martha Stewart life, before accepting that she was doing her best. Forgiving is the quickest way to shed excess weight and brings incredible lightness into your life. Do it now.

What was the one thing that when you got it, everything else seemed to fall into place?

Everything changed when I stumped up the courage to walk away from the life I was living for everyone else and accepted that I needed to speak my own truth. That was the day I started living for me.

Looking back, I can see my *raison d'être* was always to make others happy. The thought of doing something for me, I immediately labelled as selfish. It was interesting how awkward I felt at an Authentic Education session when Ben had us say, "I'm allowed" regarding living our love. He was a total stranger at the time, and I remember thinking, *Geez, why didn't I give myself permission sooner?*

I now accept my purpose in life is to live my soul's destiny, which includes helping others to live theirs.

Why do you think so many people are overwhelmed, unhappy and working in a job they dislike?

I think everyone gets caught, to a greater or lesser extent, under the rubble of societal pressures to keep up with the Joneses. They carry boulders of success *expectations*, seemingly put there by partners, family or culture. Under the layers, it's hard to hear your authentic voice, and you further disconnect from your passion. Stepping outside the status quo triggers fears and self-limiting beliefs that can keep you stuck in neutral.

I believe this is the time you need to *get naked with your authentic self*, and then go on the hunt for what *fits* you and your authentic life. You'll be less overwhelmed and happier when you're no longer shopping in another person's wardrobe. And *dahling*, trust me...you'll look *mahvelous*!

What does success mean to you?

A joyful soul is how I define success. Joy happens when you exchange a smile, feel empathy with a child or elder, see the light turn on from a lesson learned, stand in awe admiring a wondrous spectacle of nature or feel your lover's glance warm your heart. Success is never about acquiring things, but rather is a priceless feeling. It's addictive. Awareness of your soul's joy inspires you to live your truth. It keeps you on your authentic path to success. My partner always says, "Life is meant to be enjoyed, not endured." My soul totally agrees.

Why did you decide to write this chapter?

Storytelling always provides a way for humans to communicate values, lessons and possibilities. In personal transformation, I think stories about people who overcame their fears, changed their lives and are living their dreams, can provide inspiration. Writing this chapter was an absolute joy. It allowed me to articulate some of my philosophy for living and to share a bit of the story behind my business and life journey. I hope people can relate to some of our shared experiences and that I might assist connecting fellow authentic life travellers.

Connection comes in different ways for different people. You gel with some better than others. A strong connection in approach and style is the key for people to work and make magic together, whether in learning, personal transformation or social and business endeavours.

Do you have any final words?

I believe everyone can live more fully, deeply and passionately. Lose a few self-limiting beliefs, gain a few positive signposts and incrementally shift your attitude to speak your truth. Do your best, and align your life and values. Meaningful and lasting change in a short time is *totally* possible.

The sooner you start making your life better, the more enjoyment you will have. Live your dream and feed your passion, and you'll witness how your fulfilment and joy brings more love to the people around you, and the world.

You got this!

 To discover more about how *Jordan* can help you *Elevate Your Wellbeing,* simply visit www.elevatebooks.com/wellbeing

---

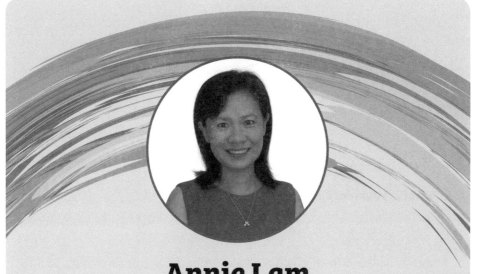

Annie Lam

Nature's Essentials

Annie Lam is a certified essential oil coach, author, speaker and educator. After finding few answers as to why her children suffered with persistent sickness, she began her quest for alternative solutions.

Upon discovering the healing power of essential oils and their use as a preventative medicine, Annie decided to become a certified essential oils coach and received a Master Aromatherapist diploma.

Annie has helped people find natural ways to improve their wellbeing and create a toxin-free home environment. She's passionate about empowering people to take a proactive approach to healthcare and enrich their lives with gentle, yet powerful, plant-based compounds.

Currently, Annie is working on her first book, *Miracles from Nature*.

For more information, please visit theessentialoilcoach.com.au

Annie Lam

Nature's Essentials

What is your most inspiring client story?

My first client was my own child.

She struggled with chronic skin issues from the age of six months and was covered with rashes and painful redness all over her face and body. We tried every product available but could never find lasting relief. Even after following a diet of immune-boosting and gut-healing foods, her skin remained inflamed.

Every doctor and dermatologist we consulted confirmed she had eczema, and their only solution was to slather her in steroid creams. You know what happened? More painful inflamed skin! No matter what we tried, her condition wasn't getting any better.

The turning point came when she was about five years old. She said to me with tears in her eyes. "Mummy, do you have a magic wand? Pleeeaaase make this go away." I felt heartbroken and helpless, since I thought I'd already done everything I could.

But guess what? This is when I finally figured out a way to make it better. I watched for synthetic chemicals in personal care products and got to work educating myself on how to make our own products using whole, natural ingredients. On our journey toward better skin, I discovered some simple, natural ingredients that did more than just smell pretty. They contained potent plant-based compounds that offered real benefits.

I applied a compress of therapeutic-grade essential oils of lavender, tea tree, frankincense and geranium, and it worked miraculously for her skin issues. I was amazed by their power and efficacy. Those tiny bottles of potion improved our life. Nine months later, her skin had fully healed. She now remains clear of eczema, and our family continues to incorporate essential oils into our life in many different ways.

What are essential oils?

Plain and simple, essential oils come from plants. They're extracted from the flower, leaves, roots, barks and peels, using steam distillation or cold pressing. To be a true essential oil, an extract must be obtained without the use of chemical solvents.

They're 75-100 times more concentrated than the oils in dried herbs. Just one drop can have powerful health benefits. For instance, it takes forty-five lemons to fill a 15ml bottle of lemon essential oil, and 8,000 roses to get a single 5ml bottle, which is about the size of your thumb.

Essential oils are volatile, meaning they evaporate readily and will pass with ease into the body. The oil's volatility is what makes it aromatic and useful in aromatherapy, since the molecules, released as vapour into the air, carry the essential oil's scent.

Keep in mind that essential oils are not a new concept. For thousands of years they've been highly prized for their healing powers and have played a key role in health and beauty rituals. There are references in the Bible to gifts of frankincense and myrrh; Hippocrates documented the effects of oils from over two-hundred herbs, and Cleopatra used rose, cypress and neroli for her beauty treatments.

However, by the 1800s pharmaceutical companies emerged, and although companies were still using plant-based medicines, synthetic drugs were gaining momentum. By the twentieth century, many people stopped using natural remedies and instead turned to convenient and effective medications offered by drug manufacturers.

Today, people are turning their attention to the actual causes of disease and away from concentrating on just making the symptoms go away. Essential oils are being rediscovered as more people look for natural ways of dealing with stress and all of its symptoms, and ensuring healthy living through diet, lifestyle and relaxation.

> "... and the leaves of the trees were for the healing of the nations." ~ Revelation 22:2

How did your family incorporate essential oils into their daily life?

Most of my earliest and significant memories have been aligned in some way to scent. As a child, I was fortunate to have my grandmother, who was enthusiastic about medicinal herbs. I remember her wearing a rounded hat, carrying a straw basket and shovel, searching for plants that would heal her aches and sores. She loved to use *Pak Fah Yeow* (white flower oil), a Chinese blend of several ingredients, including wintergreen, eucalyptus, peppermint and lavender, for easing her headaches, to clear sinus congestion and for all kinds of physical discomfort.

As a young woman, I loved exploring the sweet scents of essential oils. In the hospital during childbirth, I wanted to create a calm and relaxed environment, so I diffused lavender to reduce my anxiety. It wasn't until later, when my children were growing up, that I discovered these oils did more than smell nice. They contained powerful healing properties. My beloved grandmother was really ahead of her time!

My family now uses essential oils in extensive ways. I've used peppermint oil to repel cockroaches and bugs, clove oil to speed up the course of the flu, frankincense to quiet a migraine, lemon oil to clean my counters and herb oils in cooking.

In fact, essential oils are the first line of defence for some of the minor inconveniences usually dealt with using nasty chemicals.

This is a table of some of my family's common uses for essential oils.

Digestive relief	Peppermint, ginger, anise, fennel
Hand sanitiser	Orange, tea tree, cinnamon, rosemary, clove
Immune support	Clove, ginger, frankincense, myrrh
Menstrual Cramps	Clary sage, lavender, roman chamomile
Natural insect repellent	Lemongrass, eucalyptus, arborvitae, geranium
Non-toxic cleaner	Lemon, tea tree, lavender, orange, clove
Radiant skin	Frankincense, sandalwood, lavender, myrrh, rose
Respiratory congestion	Eucalyptus, peppermint, lemon, thyme
Restful sleep	Lavender, cedarwood, frankincense
Seasonal allergy relief	Peppermint, lemon, lavender, eucalyptus
Stress relief	Bergamot, orange, frankincense, lavender

Does toxicity play a large part in disease?

Toxicity has been known to cause problems, specifically to the central nervous system. The body has filtering systems that deal with toxins it's exposed to. However, when these systems become overloaded, toxins can accumulate in the body and lead to chronic disease.

You probably can't pronounce the names of some of the ingredients in a vast majority of personal care products. These toxic chemicals, such as preservatives, fillers and synthetic fragrances, all considered 'safe' by government standards, have been linked to multiple types of cancer, genital deformities, obesity, diabetes and infertility.

Human skin is like a sponge, and studies have confirmed that it can actually absorb seventy-five percent or more of the chemicals in any lotion or hand sanitiser.

When you become informed and understand what truly causes most diseases, you can take the necessary steps to be responsible for your own health. This is exactly what I did. Before I became an essential oil coach, I didn't have the slightest clue that the insect repellents and hand sanitisers I'd been using on my children were harming their health.

Why are essential oils so powerful?

The magic in the oils comes from chemistry.

More than just roots, stems and leaves, plants have an 'intelligence' of their own, a complicated system of communication by means of chemical messengers. These natural elements help the plant survive in its environment, influence growth and production, attract pollinating insects and repel predators. Oregano and thyme naturally ward off pathogenic bacteria, viruses and parasites, while also protecting the plant itself.

Oils can benefit your body in the same way if you suffer from infections due to the flu or common cold. This is fundamentally why essential oils are powerful as natural remedies. They contain multiple chemical constituents, which is why they have so many varied properties and uses. The healing properties of the plant are captured to restore order and balance (or homeostasis) to various bodily systems.

For instance, myrrh extract was historically used for embalming, due to its strong smell and natural antiseptic properties. But now medical scientists are finding it could be far more useful. The compound *sesquiterpenes*, obtained from myrrh, has proven to be a powerful natural substance for maintaining healthy inflammation levels in the body.

It was Rene-Maurice Gattefosse, a French chemist, who first discovered the healing properties of lavender when he severely burned his arm in a laboratory accident, immersed his hand in a vat of lavender essential oil and discovered his tissues healed quickly, without infection or scarring.

According to the National Institute of Health (NIH) PubMed database, there are currently 17,154 medical studies on essential oils, many pointing towards their therapeutic benefits and how their chemical makeup gives them power.

A lot of promising research is currently underway regarding the healing potential of essential oils in cancer patients. Frankincense (*Boswellia sacra)* has been shown to induce tumour cell death in cultured human breast cancer cells.[1] Although in-vitro research doesn't necessarily prove that a result in a lab will be as successful in the human body, it's an exciting time, and I would encourage you to keep an open mind about the possibilities for nature to boost your body's ability to heal.

"Have a mind that's open to everything and attached to nothing." ~ Dr Wayne Dyer

1 www.ncbi.nlm.nih.gov/pubmed/22171782

Here are five powerful essential oils to keep in the medicine cabinet

Essential Oil	Research	Key Benefits	Why it works
Frankincense **Boswellia**	*Boswellia frereana* extracts have been found to inhibit pro-inflammatory molecules involved in joint cartilage degradation.[1]	Boosts immunity Reduces inflammation (joints, systemic, etc) Meditation aid Minimises appearance of wrinkles & scars	**Alpha-pinene** is known for its ability to help open up the bronchial airways, making this oil useful for treating respiratory conditions.
Lavender **Lavandula angustifolia**	In human studies, lavender essential oil alleviated insomnia, anxiety and depression.[2]	First aid for burns, stings and rashes Promotes sleep Relieves headaches	**Linalyl acetate** and **linalool** have analgesic effects and are antibacterial and antiseptic.
Lemon **Citrus limon**	A study proved that lemon oil inhalation reduced nausea and vomiting during pregnancy.[3]	Uplifts the mind Non-toxic countertop spray Purifies & disinfects the air	**D-Limonene** may increase alertness and also act as a solvent.

1   Blain et al., 2009

2   www.ncbi.nlm.nih.gov/pmc/articles/PMC3612440
    https://www.unboundmedicine.com/medline/citation/22475718/Phase_II_trial_on_the_
    effects_of_Silexan_in_patients_with_neurasthenia_post_traumatic_

3   www.ncbi.nlm.nih.gov/pubmed/24829772

 Elevate Your Wellbeing

Essential Oil	Research	Key Benefits	Why it works
Peppermint *Mentha Piperita*	One study that used peppermint oil to treat irritable bowel syndrome reported an average fifty percent reduction in symptoms.[4]	Eases digestive discomfort Freshens breath Helps relieve muscle pain and headaches Food grade oils can be used for food flavouring	**Menthol** has local anaesthetic and cooling properties.
Tea Tree *Malaleuca alternifolia*	A gel with five percent tea tree oil was found to be as effective in treating acne as five percent benzoyl peroxide lotion, with fewer side effects.[5]	Cleans infections Prevents head lice Relieves cold sores Soothes dandruff	**Terpinen-4-ol** has antibacterial and antifungal properties. **Gamma-terpinene** contributes to the oil's effectiveness in fighting against infections.

---

4 https://www.ncbi.nlm.nih.gov/pubmed/17420159

5 Bassett et al., 1990

Can essential oils cure disease?

During my years of researching and reading, I've come to realise that essential oils alone won't bring someone who's in a state of disease back to healthy homeostasis. As powerful as the oils are in their effects on human beings, they're best realised when used in conjunction with a healthy lifestyle of good nutrition, regular exercise and positive thinking. Essential oils don't cure you but do boost your immune system, so your body has the tools to heal itself.

There are so many temptations in the modern world with fast food, synthetic chemicals and man-made environments. In my pursuit of healthy vitality, I seek to stay close to nature. When I eat unprocessed food that's organically grown, such as green, leafy vegetables, I remain on track with my body's vitamin and mineral needs. If I replace sweets with blueberries and kiwi fruit, I feel light and nourished. Drinking pure water from a reliable source leaves me refreshed and detoxified. Sun and fresh air provides some vitamin D, and my lungs are replenished with unpolluted oxygen.

When I use pure essential oils from the most excellent sources, such as frankincense from Somalia and tea tree from Australia, I'm offering my body, mind and spirit the finest the plant world has to offer, without being prone to damaging chemical side effects. True preventative medicine means developing good health habits using the abundant contributions of the plant world.

"The human body has the power to heal itself—it just needs a little bit of help from nature." ~ Rudolf Steiner

What are the modern methods for using essential oils?

ESSENTIAL OIL THERAPY

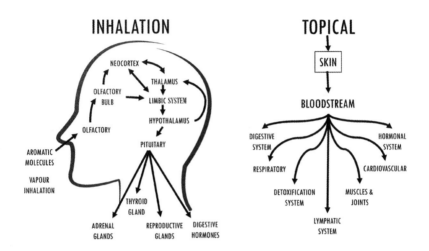

Inhalation

Inhaling certain essential oils can change the way you feel almost instantly. They're quickly absorbed by the smell receptors, which have a direct link to the limbic system by way of the olfactory nerve. The limbic system is the part of the brain that supports a variety of functions, including smell, emotions, behaviour and memory.

In fact, research shows that the symptoms of everything from nausea, stress, and insomnia, to anxiety disorders, dementia, and high blood pressure, can be reduced.

Some of the benefits of inhaling essential oils include:

▸ Enhancing memory and concentration

Researchers have found that essential oil from rosemary enhances memory by 60-75 percent compared with people who had not been exposed to it. But while rosemary essential oil is generally regarded as *the* oil to use for memory and concentration, lemon and peppermint essential oils can also be helpful in staying focused and alert.

Shakespeare said, "There's rosemary, that's for remembrance..."

▸ Stimulating the smell receptors

A cold air diffuser filled with a blend of lavender, tangerine and cedarwood, can be used to give your living room a homey fragrance.

▸ Remedying a cold through steam inhalation

Add a drop each of eucalyptus, peppermint and tea tree into a bowl of steaming hot water, sit directly in front of it and cover your head and bowl with a towel.

When you inhale essential oils, they enter your respiratory system and cross your blood-brain barrier. In your lungs, molecules of essential oils attach to oxygen molecules and are carried into your bloodstream, where they're circulated to every cell in your body. Within the cells, essential oils can activate healing and improve your health and wellbeing.

Topical

Essential oils are absorbed effectively through the skin.

You can rub them directly onto your neck or feet for a feeling of relaxation. For example, applying lavender to the temples and the back of the neck can help get you into a relaxed state of rejuvenation.

TIP: *Before attempting these methods, you need to dilute the essential oils because of the high concentration of compounds they contain. The way you do this is with carrier oils. They reduce the risk of skin sensitivity from topical application and provide soothing comfort should irritation or redness occur. Vegetable oils make up the bulk of carrier oils used in aromatherapy.*

Even when diluted, the oils will still have a strong healing effect.

Essential oils have the ability to penetrate the skin's surface through pores and hair follicles and work from the inside, where they're absorbed by the capillaries. Once in the bloodstream, they can affect adjacent organs and structures and circulate throughout the entire body to restore balance.

Unlike synthetic drugs, essential oils don't accumulate in the body and have a low potential to be physically habit-forming, because they're eliminated quickly through the skin and organs.

Culinary Uses

Food grade essential oils can be used in low doses for applications such as cooking, flavouring, mouth washes and throat sprays. Adding a few drops of essential oils to your food or beverage will highlight a special flavour. For instance, you can add a drop of peppermint oil in raw chocolate slices, lemon oil in homemade gummy jellies, or oregano oil in spaghetti sauce. They not only enhance the flavour, but you get all of the healthful benefits from the oil.

Only use food grade oils marked as a dietary supplement. Not all essential oils are created equal, and most on the market aren't safe to be ingested. Also, they're super concentrated, so start out with only using one drop.

TIP: *As essential oils are highly potent, it's recommended you consult a healthcare professional before ingesting therapeutic doses.*

Are there safety considerations when using essential oils?

Essential oils are natural. However, they're highly concentrated, so you need some safety guidelines to follow to guarantee safe and effective use.

- Check with a qualified health practitioner before using essential oils, or any other remedy, especially if you are pregnant or have a health condition.

- Select only the highest quality oils that are 100% pure and sourced from the country where the plant is indigenous.

- Choose a brand that offers third-party GC/MS testing reports to ensure there are no harmful substances such as pesticides, toxins, fragrances and fillers.

- Most essential oils require prior mixing with a carrier oil, such as fractionated coconut oil, to dilute the concentration and prevent skin irritation. Some carrier oils are more suitable than others due to the size of the molecule and are more readily absorbed.

- Don't use in the eyes or inside ear canals.

- Discontinue use if you experience any irritation or discomfort.

- When treating children, do a skin sensitivity test with a small amount and follow dilution guidelines.

- Some citrus oils can cause a phototoxic skin reaction when applied topically. Avoidance of sunlight is recommended for up to twelve hours after use.

- Less is more, and consistency is key! Even though essential oils are 'natural', keep in mind that they are potent, and a little goes a long way.

TIP: Make sure the oils you buy have the botanical (Latin) name of the plant on the bottle. This helps to ensure it's actually an essential oil, rather than a synthetically manufactured fragrance oil. There are some plants that are known by more than one botanical name, and they don't necessarily share the same therapeutic properties or benefits.

As always, see a healthcare professional if symptoms persist or worsen.

What courses have you taken that enabled you to get started or build your business?

I definitely didn't plan on getting into natural health. It was a business that started itself.

I was a mum pursuing my own career in the area of accounting and taxation. Children are extremely precious, and as a parent, you're the first responder when it comes to their health and wellbeing. When they get sick, you want to do everything in your power to make them feel better. But when your actions don't provide relief, it can be a frustrating experience.

I never dreamed two decades ago, when I graduated from the University of Sydney with a Bachelor in Commerce, that I would ever be educating and empowering people about how to integrate safer and more effective solutions for their family's health.

I'm also a qualified member of The Chartered Accountants in Australia and New Zealand (CAANZ), and I used that same training to research articles on natural health and essential oil science.

It wasn't until I received more formal education during my studies with the Australian College of Aromatherapy, as well as with the Essential Oil Institute of America, that I really learnt how to dig deep into the science that makes essential oils so powerful. I was blown away by what I discovered.

In sharing my journey with others, I realised that a lot of families were interested in how natural remedies could help support the health and wellbeing of themselves and their loved ones.

Do you have a coach or mentor to motivate you?

When I was researching everything I could regarding food, nutrition and natural personal care, I came across some fabulous natural health practitioners. Although I haven't met them in person, they ignited my passion for living a holistic lifestyle.

Dr Josh Axe talked about using therapeutic-grade essential oils to heal various skin conditions, such as my daughter's. I was sceptical at first, but my worries ceased once her skin started getting better. I've been there. I know what it feels like when your children are constantly unwell. Helping my children on their journey to health crystallised my life mission.

I'm also grateful to Gwendoline Ford, principal at the Australian College of Aromatherapy, and her team, as they gave me tremendous support and motivation during my aromatherapy studies. Gwendoline is a renowned leader in the natural health industry.

Dr Natasha Campbell-McBride and her book, *Gut and Psychology Syndrome*, have been invaluable to me. I learnt about the link between what you eat and drink and the condition of the digestive system. Some health sources claim that eighty percent of the immune system exists in the gut, so I began feeding my children nutritious broths and probiotic-rich fermented vegetables, and they've become so much healthier.

What are you passionate about?

I'm passionate about sharing my knowledge regarding natural alternatives to the current toxic cocktail of products and health practices, and reminding people to be mindful of what they apply topically onto, and ingest into, their body.

One of the best and most rewarding parts of my life is paying forward all that I've learned. When you feel the time is right, reach out to me. I would be glad to help show you the way.

Why is health important?

Material objects come and go, but without good health, you wouldn't be able to live a fulfilling life. By taking care of yourself and maintaining a healthy lifestyle, you will:

- look and feel better
- be more productive
- be more confident and ready to take on challenges
- have more energy
- be more emotionally stable

"A person who has their health has a thousand dreams. A person who does not, has just one." ~ Unknown

What are the best ways people can have more energy?

Everyone struggles with some sort of fatigue or exhaustion. And of course, being tired is normal when it gets late in the evening and you're going through a stressful time in your life.

But being chronically tired is not normal, and many people today struggle from adrenal fatigue, which occurs when the body and adrenal glands can't keep up with prolonged daily or chronic stress. Common symptoms include weight gain, insomnia, body aches, trouble concentrating, constantly feeling tired, hormone imbalance, reduced sex drive and food cravings.

The best way I've found to boost my energy naturally and overcome adrenal issues is by soaking in a nice, warm healing bath at night with chamomile and vetiver oils, and Epsom salts. In some medical studies, chamomile has been shown to reduce gut inflammation, but it's also good for adrenals, because it helps calm a tense nervous system.

People with adrenal fatigue have a heightened or hyperactive sympathetic nervous system. They live in the fight-or-flight response, and it's critical to break that cycle. This method is a great healing therapy and helps you sleep well.

"A perfumed bath and a scented massage every day is the way to good health" ~ Hippocrates

How can someone improve their health and wellbeing?

If you're in search of a healthy and vibrant life, you should focus your energy on preventing disease before it ever takes root in your body. For instance, I really used to believe that if I focused on one thing, like eating a super-healthy diet, I'd be cured. But what I found is that it's a combination of a lot of different techniques; the whole package of eating right, getting sleep and eliminating stress, and adding these natural remedies of plant-based products, do a wonderful job of aiding in your total wellbeing.

The Five Steps of Wellbeing pyramid:

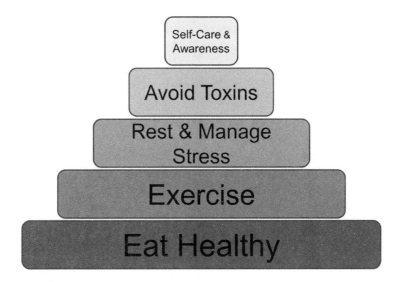

Self-Care & Awareness

Avoid Toxins

Rest & Manage Stress

Exercise

Eat Healthy

Eat Healthy

Your diet should be rich in foods with an abundance of antioxidants, vitamins, minerals and enzymes. Choose fresh, unprocessed food that comes from nature, and avoid refined sugars, preservatives, chemicals, pesticides and added hormones.

Exercise

Regular, moderate exercise is important for physical and emotional wellness. It begins with taking the stairs, walking to the shops and generally having a mentality of movement. A complete exercise program can include strength, aerobic and flexibility training.

Rest and Manage Stress

Your body needs appropriate time for rest and relaxation for a healthy immune system. Getting a good night's sleep is essential, and so is practicing relaxation techniques for optimal health.

Avoid Toxins

Every day you're exposed to environmental stressors, such as pollutants in the air and water, harmful ingredients and electro-magnetic fields. Being aware of these threats, and choosing non-toxic products, are important factors to obtaining optimal health.

Self-care and awareness

Your primary duty is to protect your family, and most importantly, think for yourself and take control of your own health. Focus on more proactive measures of preventing disease, and work towards boosting your immune system.

What makes people medicate with drugs and other substances?

It's a known fact that medicinal drugs have negative side-effects. For every benefit they offer, there's a disadvantage for the body. However, people still take them on a regular basis, because they offer quick relief from pain and reduce inflammation.

Although tests have proven that aspirin can irritate the stomach lining and cause liver damage, people take them and believe they're safe. These pills only mask symptoms and don't get to the root cause of the disease, which is some kind of imbalance in the body, so it's going to come back.

My children had a weakened immune system and were always coming down with infections. They also struggled with digestive issues and food sensitivities, and we took medications on an ongoing basis for every minor illness. This went on for years and years, because we lived in that medical mindset. I've learnt that overusing these medications can cause micronutrient deficiencies, which essentially creates other issues within the body.

For example, antibiotics are used for infections, because they kill bacteria. However, there are good bacteria living in your body, without which it can't work efficiently. As a result, many people suffer illnesses such as irritable bowel syndrome, food allergies and other intolerances. Also, whenever antibiotics are used, the body builds up resistance to them, which means stronger doses are needed to fight infections, and the cycle continues.

A report issued by the World Health Organisation (WHO) has validated what many holistic health experts have been suggesting for years: overuse of antibiotics causes drug resistance and puts the globe at risk of superbugs. These are micro-organisms (bacteria, fungus or virus) that are immune to drugs and have the potential to literally become invincible.

Many essential oils are antiseptic and act as natural antibiotics against viruses, fungi and bacteria. Their complexity prevents the development of resistance, a major concern with prescription drugs. Although modern medicine does have its place in health care, greater preference should be given to the least invasive option that can still effectively remedy the problem.

It the benefits of a drug outweigh its risks, or if it's necessary to preserve life, it becomes a viable option. Conversely, if a natural option is available that will serve the same purpose as the drug, but with less risk, it should be the first choice to consider. I believe that applying this principle protects public health and may reverse the unfavourable trend of using drugs for every ailment.

> "Cure by food is better than cure by medicine"
> ~ Chinese Saying

What's one thing someone could do now to change their life?

I encourage you to take personal responsibility for your life and health.

It's imperative that you take preventative measures to stay healthy, such as eating better and exercising.

I took personal responsibility by doing my research and making sure we had quality food in our refrigerator. Remember that every time you put something in your mouth, your body takes those nutrients, or lack thereof, to build or break down your cells.

Do you have any last words to share?

I wholeheartedly believe the solution to many health problems are found in nature. It's important to remove the toxins that invade your body through your food, water, personal care products and cleaning supplies, and replace these conventional approaches with innovations specifically designed to restore health.

 To discover more about how *Annie* can help you *Elevate Your Wellbeing,* simply visit www.elevatebooks.com/wellbeing

---

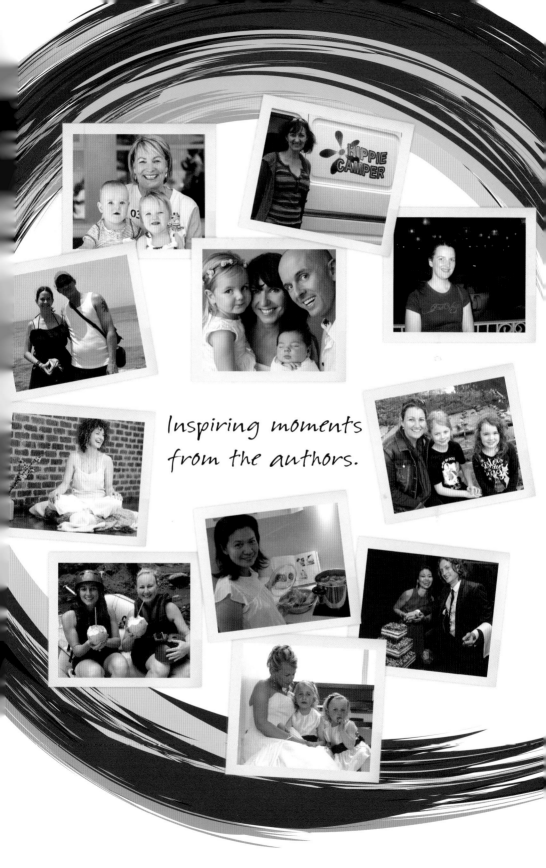

Inspiring moments from the authors.

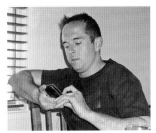

Ben in his 'larger' not-so-healthy days.

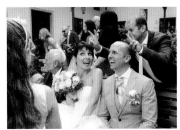

Ben and his wife on their wedding day in a castle in the Czech Republic.

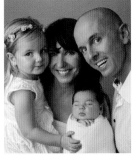

Ben with his wife Marketa and daughters Annabella and Jasmine.

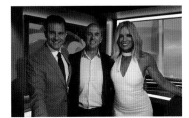

Ben on set after one of his live interviews for the Today Show on Channel 9, with hosts David Campbell and Sonia Kruger.

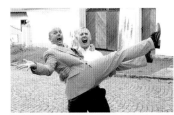

Ben with his Dad.

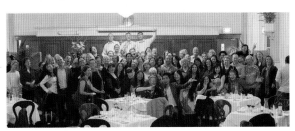

Ben taking his students to dinner upstairs at Authentic Education Academy in Sydney, located inside of a boutique hotel.

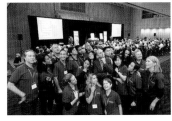

Benjamin Harvey, Cham Tang and Toni Neill (Crew Director and Events Manager), with the crew in blue at an Authentic Education event.

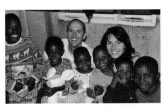

Ben and his wife donating bunk beds and toys at an orphanage in Tanzania.

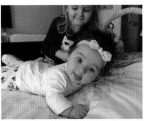

Ben's daughters, Jasmine and Annabella.

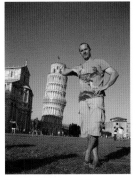

Ben doing the obligatory Leaning Tower of Pisa pose.

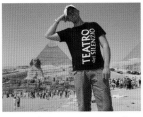

Benjamin Harvey on vacation in Egypt.

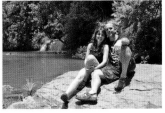

Ben and Marketa on holiday in Cuba.

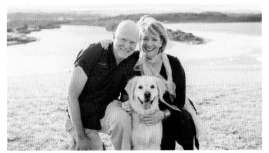

Heather and her husband sharing the great outdoors with Sasha the therapy dog.

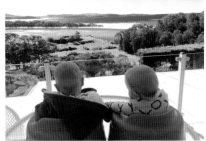

Heather's twin grandchildren soaking up the view from her home, where she runs Marriage Getaways.

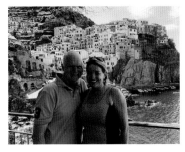

Heather and her husband hiking in Cinque Terre, Italy.

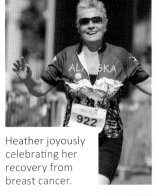

Heather joyously celebrating her recovery from breast cancer.

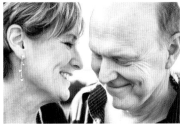

Heather running in the 2018 Commonwealth Games Baton Relay.

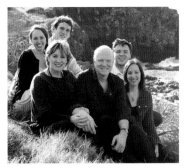

Heather with her husband, John, sharing a connecting moment.

Heather and her family by the ocean.

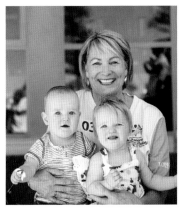

Heather celebrating the joy of grandchildren.

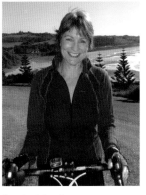

Fundraising for cancer research by cycling from Sydney to Mt. Kosciuszko.

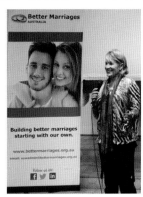

Heather presenting a seminar to help people strengthen their relationships.

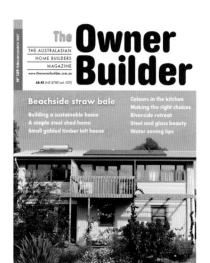

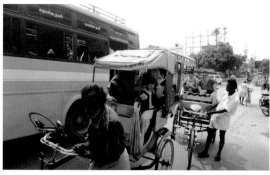

Tina in a cycle rickshaw in India.

The cover of Owner- Builder magazine, featuring the beachside strawbale house Tina Bolto built.

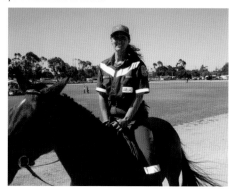

Tina Bolto on paramedic duty at the Pinnaroo show.

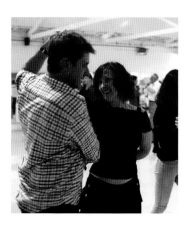

Tina at an afternoon tea dance party.

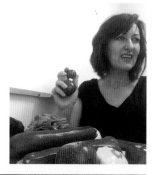

Tina Bolto teaching with some of her produce.

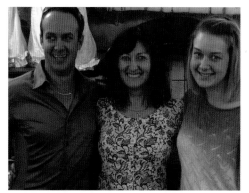

Tina with her (now adult) children, Adam and Kerry-Lee.

Tina taking a road trip from Sydney to Cairns.

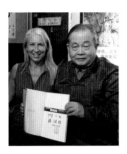

Jordan Alexander meeting the last living farmer, who was one of three people to discover the archaeological wonder of China's first Emperor QinShihuang, which is now part of the world-renowned twenty hectare Terracotta Museum.

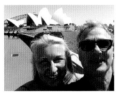

Jordan with the love of her life, Rick, on holiday in Sydney.

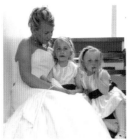

Jordan enjoying some quiet time on her big day with two of her biggest successes in life, her daughters Sage and Ella.

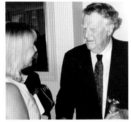

Jordan at NZ Government House meeting her hero, Sir Edmund Hillary, the first person to climb Mt Everest, who said, "It's not the mountain we conquer, but ourselves".

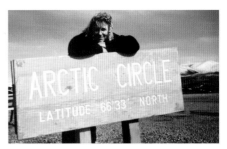

Listening to the call of the Great White North, Jordan Alexander travels to Alaska and the Arctic Circle.

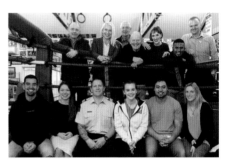

The Billy Graham Youth Foundation using boxing and good old-fashioned values like respect to make a difference with at-risk youths throughout Aotearoa. Photographer: Robert Cross

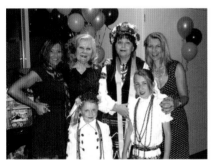

Jordan Alexander enjoying New Zealand's Maori culture in Northland, Aotearoa on her first visit from Canada.

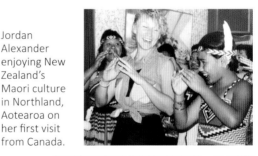

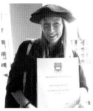

Jordan's mum, Tatiana (two from left), with her daughters and grand-daughters, celebrating her seventieth birthday and their Ukrainian heritage.

Jordan is all smiles as she becomes a graduate of the University of Auckland.

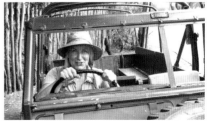

Jordan Alexander, having fun at the Wellington Zoo, while filming her YouTube video, *Ten Tips for Online Dating*.

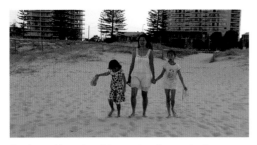

Annie and her daughters going for a relaxing walk at the beach.

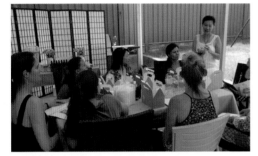

Annie presenting at one of her events.

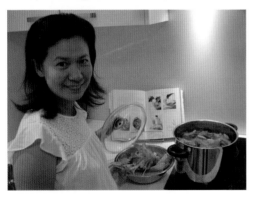

Annie cooking up nutritious and gut-healing chicken bone broth.

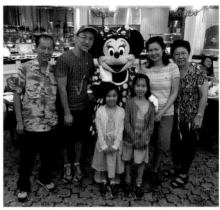

Family trip to Disneyland in Hong Kong.

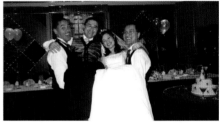

Annie and her husband, Charles, clowning around on their wedding day.

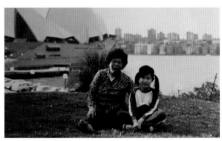

Little Annie spending time with her beloved grandmother.

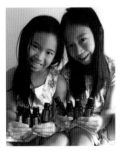

Annie's daughters, Ashleigh and Jessica, displaying their favourite essential oils.

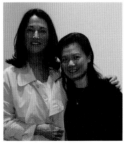

Annie at the Therese Kerr's Inner Origin event about living a chemical-free lifestyle.

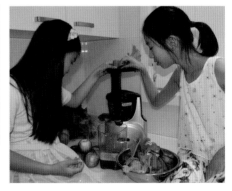

Annie's girls making freshly squeezed juice!

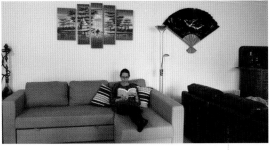

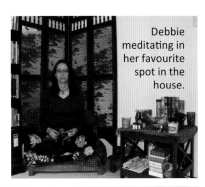

Debbie meditating in her favourite spot in the house.

Debbie engaging in one of her favourite pastimes: reading.

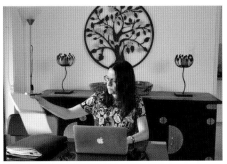

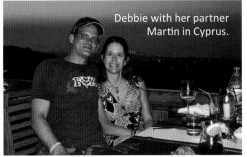

Debbie with her partner Martin in Cyprus.

Debbie hard at work on her next book.

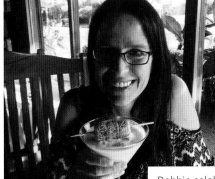

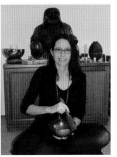

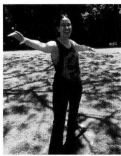

Debbie practicing with one of her Tibetan singing bowls.

Who said yoga's hard work?

Debbie celebrating the completion of her EFT training course with a marshmallow vodka cocktail.

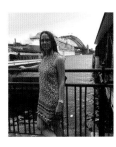

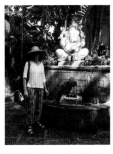

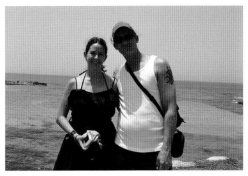

First visit to Circular Quay, shortly after arriving in Sydney from London.

Debbie about to head out for a walk during a Balinese yoga retreat.

Debbie on holiday with her partner, Martin.

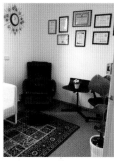
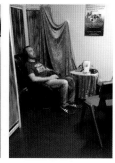
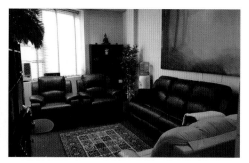

This was Bridget's first office when she gained the confidence to start her own hypnotherapy business.

Gavin O'Neill was one of Bridget's first clients at the wellness festival.

Bridget needed a bigger space to treat quit smoking and weight loss groups.

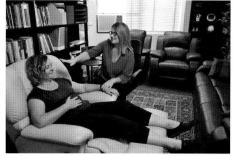

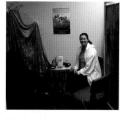
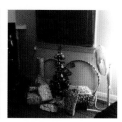

Having the courage to participate in a wellness festival got Bridget's career up and running.

Bridget's first Christmas back in Australia was tight, but they were grateful for the roof over their heads.

Bridget performing hypnosis on one of her clients, Rachel Dunn, to help her quit smoking.

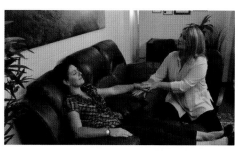

Bridget performing hypnosis on one of her clients, Rebecca Nehme, at her clinic in Parramatta.

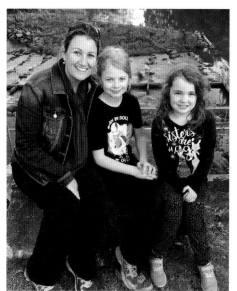

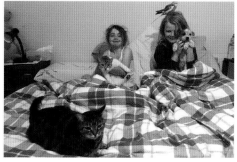

Bridget with her two children, Matilda and Eleanor, enjoying the outdoors.

Bridget's children having fun with their adorable pets.

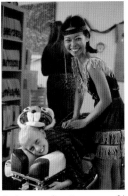

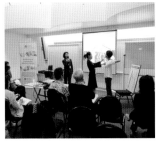

Dr Irene after completing her first half marathon run in 2014.

Dr Irene doing a demonstration at a community talk on how to prevent back pain.

Dr Irene adjusting one of her clients at Be Chiropractic's annual Kid's day.

Dr Irene and her staff at Be Chiropractic's children's Christmas party.

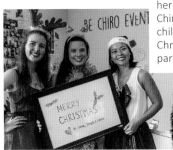

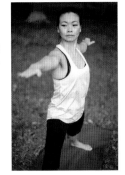

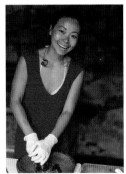

Yoga is a big part of Dr Irene's exercise regime.

Dr Irene learning how to cook Thai cuisine in Thailand.

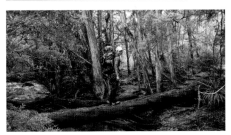

Dr Irene getting in touch with nature while hiking Cradle Mountain.

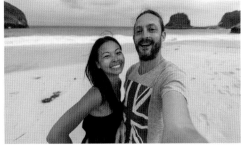

Dr Irene enjoying a beach holiday in Lombok with her husband.

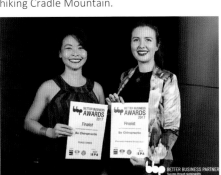

Dr Irene Chin proudly displaying her two Better Business finalist awards for Be Chiropractic in 2017.

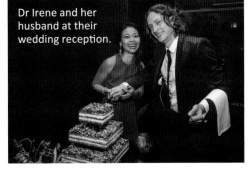

Dr Irene and her husband at their wedding reception.

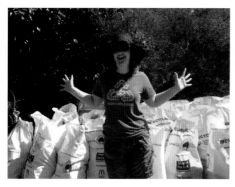

Gretchen taking part in Clean-up Australia Day in 2016.

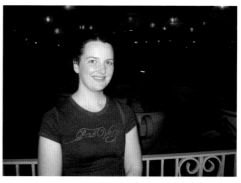

Gretchen at Disneyland in California in 2011.

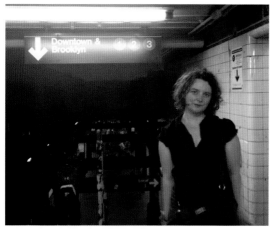

Gretchen taking the subway in New York in 2015.

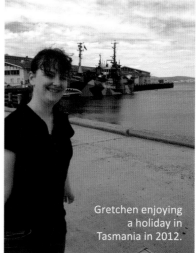

Gretchen enjoying a holiday in Tasmania in 2012.

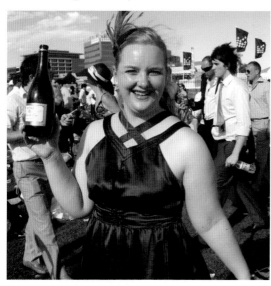

Gretchen at the Spring Racing Carnival in Melbourne in 2008.

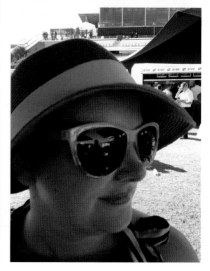

Gretchen at the Melbourne Cup in 2013.

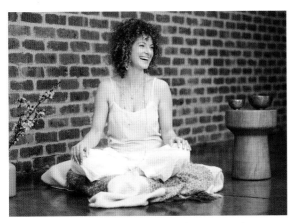

Deborah loves mindful practices, including yoga and meditation.

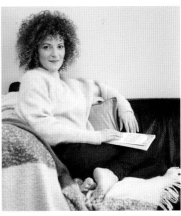

Deborah reading about the mind-soul-body connection.

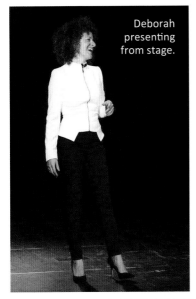

Deborah presenting from stage.

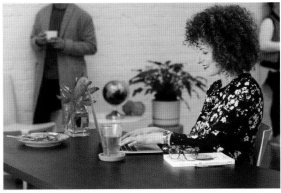

Deborah creating programs that help people live rich, full and meaningful lives.

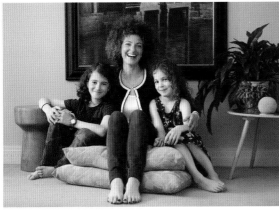

Deborah with her son and daughter.

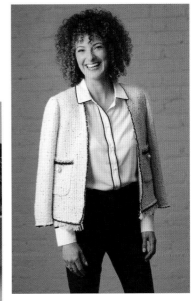

Deborah at a mastermind event in Melbourne.

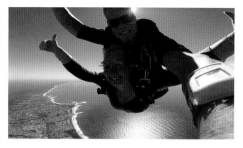

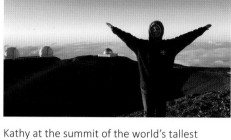

Kathy indulging her enjoyment of adrenalin sports, skydiving on the beach of Wollongong in NSW.

Kathy at the summit of the world's tallest mountain, Mauna Kea, in Hawaii.

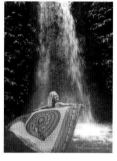

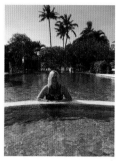

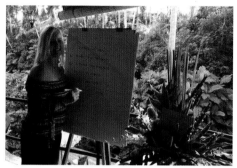

Kathy enjoying her love of waterfalls in Bali.

Kathy relaxing in Northern Bali at a resort where she holds retreats.

Kathy Morrison presenting a workshop at her Women's Retreat in Ubud, Bali.

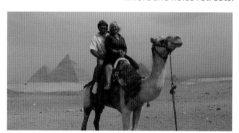

Kathy and her husband, Peter, on a camel ride at the Pyramids of Giza in Egypt.

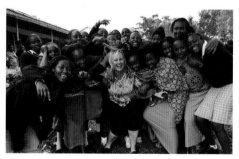

Kathy visiting a secondary orphanage school in Kenya, where the teenagers had a fascination with her blonde hair.

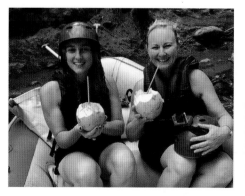

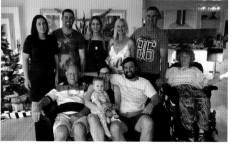

Kathy and her daughter, Megan, enjoying a coconut after taking on the white water rapids of Bali.

Kathy with her family on Christmas Day in 2016.

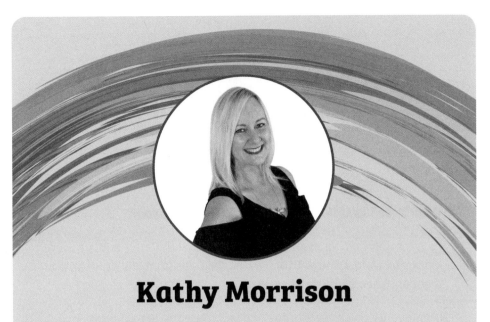

Kathy Morrison

Passion, Travel and Freedom

Kathy Morrison is a certified life coach and women's retreat facilitator.

The freedom to travel the world, go on adventures and do what she loves, inspires her to take women on an unforgettable journey of learning, self-discovery, transformation and connecting to other cultures.

Kathy's holistic approach to life, and her belief in alternative therapies, led her to study the ancient self-healing power of crystals and shamanic teachings, as well as become a practitioner of Australian Bush Flower Essences.

For thirty years, Kathy has been a carer for her daughter, Jenna, who has a profound disability. This experience has taught her that through life's challenges, there's always the ability to change, accomplish the possible and enjoy an authentic and passionate life.

Kathy Morrison

Passion, Travel and Freedom

What's the worst thing that's ever happened to you?

I'd been married for two years to my husband, Peter, and we were looking forward to the birth of our first child after a previous miscarriage that happened at fourteen weeks.

I was twenty-three years of age and had the world at my feet, when my life changed. I went down a different path, one I never dreamt I'd be living and ultimately had no control over.

On the 17th of July 1987, I gave birth to my daughter, Jenna. I was so excited about meeting my first child and took for granted that this would be a time of pure happiness and joy. But for the first week of Jenna's life, she was critically ill and struggling to survive.

Living in the country and being a great distance from a major hospital meant that having an ill newborn baby was a terrifying experience.

Jenna had to immediately be transported to a larger hospital. Since there was a risk she would pass away before they reached their destination, her nurse had to baptise her in the back of the ambulance.

I was exhausted from the birth and terrified. Feeling numb and overwhelmed, I thought that if she died, I wanted to die, too. I didn't get the opportunity to hold or bond with her, which greatly distressed me, and I felt robbed of that first nurturing experience as a mother. My heart was breaking, but there wasn't a thing I could do other than pray she would survive.

Two days later I was well enough to travel, so my husband and I flew to Camperdown Children's Hospital in Sydney. When we got there, we didn't know whether she'd be alive or not.

What I witnessed that day, when I walked into the neonatal intensive care unit, is etched in my mind forever. A tiny newborn fighting for her life. My baby was attached to so many tubes on her tiny body, that it was shocking to even look at. I was broken but trying so hard to be brave and not cry. Each morning I'd wake up and be thankful I hadn't received a phone call during the night telling me she'd deteriorated. Every day I would walk through the big old doors of the hospital, not knowing whether my daughter was alive.

Jenna did survive her birth trauma and came home to live with us when she was a month old, but only four months later she was diagnosed with profound cerebral palsy. This life event was the start of a difficult journey as a parent and carer of a child with a major disability. It's impacted our lives in every aspect for the last thirty years.

They say what doesn't kill you makes you stronger. Those life lessons have made me the person I am today and given me the passion to inspire others who are experiencing adversity on their life journey.

How have your life experiences changed you?

As a result of the constant twenty-four-hour care needs of my daughter and three more beautiful children, I was struggling to cope as a mother and wife, which led to the deterioration of my health. My life was spiralling out of control as I dealt with depression, anxiety and panic attacks, and I found it difficult to leave the house. Since I was a teenager, I'd suffered from perfectionism and Obsessive Compulsive Disorder (OCD), which robbed me of enjoying my life with my family.

Then, five years ago I decided it was time to look at ways to improve my mental and emotional health and find my authentic self. Due to the daily pressures of caring for my family, I'd lost my identity and had no self-worth. I was negative about life in general, angry and constantly dealing with fear-based problems, as well as judgment of others.

Through my own journey of self-development, I rediscovered who I really was. I found the freedom to do what I love and live my life to the fullest. As a fulltime carer, I led a different life from most and missed out on so many life experiences.

By thinking outside of the box and constantly challenging my thoughts, behaviours and actions, I started to believe that life can be anything you want it to be if you're determined and willing to try, despite the obstacles put in your path. I learnt to take each day as it comes and that it's impossible to be happy one-hundred percent of the time.

Once I came to realise that I could change my mindset and how I react to negative outcomes, I started to see the joy in the simple things in life. I challenged myself to learn something new each day, wrote a bucket list of what I'd always wanted to do and slowly realised those dreams as I accomplished them. It gave my life meaning, purpose and happiness.

I also realised that to express gratitude for my many blessings, I needed to give back and be of service by helping others on their journey.

Have you had any aha moments that changed everything for you?

Five years ago I was given the opportunity to travel with friends to Europe on an adventure that took me to six countries in six weeks: France, Italy, Turkey, Egypt, Santorini in the Greek islands, Athens and Dubai in The United Arab Emirates.

I never thought I would be able to travel overseas, as my daughter required fulltime care. But through extensive planning, support and help from others around me, I was able to embark on an adventure that changed my life and how I viewed the world.

My travelling experiences become my teacher. Learning about different cultures gave new meaning and joy to my life.

Where you reside is only a drop in the ocean of the world you live in.

What this experience taught me is that if you put your mind to something and believe in yourself, you can accomplish anything and overcome the adversity that's holding you back from exploring your best life. It was an important lesson to learn.

Always remember to ask yourself, *What else is possible?*

What courses have you taken that enabled you to get started or build your business?

▶ My holistic approach to health led me to study how to balance the mind, body and soul for ultimate wellness.

▶ I have a background working with women in nutrition and fitness, which included weight management programming, as well as speaking, mentoring and coaching.

▶ I've taken mind-based courses in Queensland and The Mind Detox Academy in Sydney.

▶ I've achieved Level 1 in Vibrational Kinesiology for alternative healing of the body.

▶ I've completed Level 1 and 2 in Australian Bush Flower Vibrational Healing Essences.

- I have an advanced diploma in Crystal Shamanism Training in Australia, Bali and Hawaii. This method of alternative medicine is the ancient wisdom of healing the body energetically with crystals.

- I became an Authentic Education Certified Life Coach, which gives me the opportunity to help others be the best version of themselves.

- I've gone through the Authentic Education PHD program, which includes five core areas: business, marketing, public speaking, wealth creation and success automation.

- I received extensive training with Vibrant Women in Bali to become a women's retreat facilitator, so I can help women travel to wonderful places around the world.

How did you become interested in being a retreat facilitator?

I'd always liked the idea of going on a retreat. It offers a different learning perspective and environment than a classroom, with the added advantage of travel, experiencing different cultures and exploring the surroundings areas.

I started in self-development, which included mind-based training, and I'd been on several retreats over the years in Australia and Bali as part of those trainings. I then had shamanic training in Bali and Hawaii, where I gained experience regarding different styles of retreats.

My certified life coach training taught me a broad range of teaching tools to incorporate into retreats. I wanted to have a career doing what I was passionate about, so taking what I love to do, which is having fun while empowering and changing women's lives, and blending it with my love of travel and culture, seemed like a good idea.

I have what I like to call The Ten R's of retreating.

1. **Retreat:** Escape the world

2. **Recognise:** Understand your need to be nurtured, so you can sustain yourself and others

3. **Relax**: Calm your body, mind and approach to life

4. **Revitalise**: Slow down, breathe deeply and sleep soundly

5. **Restore**: Reinvigorate your sense of balance and equanimity

6. **Replenish:** Renew your strength, vitality and energy for life

7. **Release**: Let go of your expectations and just be

8. **Reflect**: Contemplate your purpose and the meaning of your life

9. **Renew**: Find a new perspective on life

10. **Rejoice:** Have fun, and celebrate all that you are

What do you offer with your women's retreats?

I'm a woman's retreat facilitator and lover of life, so I want to inspire other women by taking them on an unforgettable voyage to exotic and beautiful places around the world.

I believe it's important to feel the true essence of what other cultures have to offer, while residing in comfortable accommodation and having your specific dietary needs catered to. These retreats focus on:

- personal development

- forming friendships

- connecting with like-minded women

- bonding as a sisterhood

- supporting and encouraging one another

- pampering

- shopping

- having fun

This adventure is also for those women leading a chaotic, stressful and overwhelming life, who want to get away to have some quality downtime while having their needs met.

There's time to reflect, relax and rejuvenate. We have yoga and meditation, as well as spiritual experiences, such as visiting your own medicine man in Bali as in the movie *Eat, Pray, Love!* You can also participate in cultural activities like a cooking class where you indulge in making yummy culinary delights that are literally food for the soul.

All retreats are custom designed to be a life-changing experience that's aligned with the location. For instance, they can be tailored for small get-togethers, a special occasion like a milestone birthday or a girls-just-wanna-have-fun weekend.

There are also packages available for corporate team building.

Here's what's included:

▶ Connection with another culture

▶ Rejuvenation of the soul and time for self-reflection

▶ A journey of self-discovery through mindfulness and transformation life-coaching

- Gaining an understanding that it's never too late to live your dream life

- Pampering , spa treatments and massage

- Free time to relax and explore

- Guided direction and support to achieve a mindset change

- Learning how to take risks and allowing yourself to step out of your comfort zone

- Discovering how to be a free spirit and that anything is possible

- Cooking classes

- Food and wine experiences

- An opportunity to build new authentic friendships through this community

- Fun, laughter, bonding and nurturing with other women in amazing places

- Cultural and spiritual activities

- Workshops

- Learning how to have confidence and self-love

- Optional adrenaline and adventure activities, such as:

  - trekking

  - white water rafting

  - sky diving

- paragliding

- parasailing

- jet skiing

- snorkelling

- quad biking

Why is mindset Important?

Your mindset influences the way you live your life. It's the basic foundation for how you think, act and feel. Values and beliefs, childhood conditioning, life experiences and emotions and behaviours are all influenced by your mindset. This is why I love retreats. In this environment, I can challenge women with different mindsets to change their perception and quality of life by embracing other environments, travel opportunities and learning models. In this way, they can understand how to live a fun and expansive life and reach their true potential.

Live your dreams. "Change your thinking, change your life."

What's the one message you wish to share with the world?

Life is too short to live the same day twice. Never be afraid to get out of your comfort zone and challenge yourself, because that's where the real magic happens.

Some of your best achievements are on the other side of fear. I've accomplished many life-changing experiences by the motto, "Feel the fear, and do it anyway."

What is the ultimate life lesson?

Learning to accept what you cannot change.

When I realised my daughter would never get to reach her full potential, after all of the hopes and dreams I had for her and what could have been, I was devastated. I struggled with comparing her to other children while watching them reach their milestones. It was difficult not to feel ripped off for my daughter, who carried the burden of a 'disabled' identity, due to her profound cerebral palsy. There was an overwhelming sense of grief and loss. To not have a 'normal' family doing 'normal' things was too much for my mind to overcome, and I often wondered why this had to happen to me.

It had an impact on my marriage and our other three children as they grew up, but we did the best we could with the difficult family structure. We all became more compassionate to the needs of those who were less fortunate, while receiving some valuable life lessons.

But at one point I dug deep to realise how lucky I was and became thankful for having my precious family to fill my heart with joy. I became grateful for all that I did have and fought long and hard to make my life what it is today. I discovered that the mind is a powerful tool, and when you use it, you can achieve great things. Most People don't realise how powerfully strong you can be through adversity, until you're challenged to the max.

From early on, the mantra I repeated to myself each morning was, "I choose to swim and not sink." I fought the currents that were trying to drown me and my spirit, rose above feeling overwhelmed and conquered my demons. The eagle is now my totem and I wear it around my neck as a representation of my shamanic journey of healing and who I've become. My motto is *First Love Yourself*, so I like to say I FLY like an Eagle. Nothing touches the eagle. It rises above all and represents my freedom to live my life the way I want.

What does being spiritual mean to you?

▸ Having more depth, caring and awareness of the world.

▸ Experiencing a greater level of consciousness for all we do and how we think and feel.

▸ Realising there's something great and powerful in the universe that can't be explained.

▸ Asking the universe for what you need, being open to receiving it and setting intentions to manifest goals.

Do you have any words of wisdom to share?

▸ The world is your oyster, so make your life what you want it to be. When you're challenged, know there are always ways you can improve your current situation.

▸ Each day you're alive is a blessing, and you must find happiness and joy in the small things like a walk on the beach, the sun rising and setting, the grass under your feet, listening to music and a conversation with a friend.

▸ Be grateful for all you have, and live each day as though it's your last.

▸ Everything happens for a reason, but you may not understand it at the time.

▸ Anything is possible if you dream big.

▸ Be true to yourself and what you believe in.

▸ Live in the present, and be mindful of all you do.

▸ When women support each other, incredible things happen.

▸ Never stop learning, because life never stops teaching.

▸ Travel and learn about other cultures. It will enrich your life experiences.

Why do you think so many people feel overwhelmed and unhappy?

Many people's lives are out of balance. They're time poor and stuck with no purpose or direction, because they're far too busy doing activities that aren't important instead of doing what they love.

What they should be focusing on is creating a balanced mindset, so they can improve their life and wellbeing. This can be achieved by focusing on their thoughts, behaviours, habits and outlook on life.

People need to get back to basics and live a more simple life.

How would you like to be remembered?

I would like to be remembered as a free-spirited, strong woman who after overcoming her own life struggles, helped inspire and empower others to live their life with purpose, be adventurous, explore life outside the box and overcome their fears in order to reach their full potential.

What do you think your life purpose is?

Helping people overcome adversities through transformational life coaching, travel, retreats and cultural experiences around the world.

If you were speaking to your younger self, what advice would you give?

I would look deeply into her eyes, put my hand on her heart and say:

▸ Life is a series of many lessons. Accept and acknowledge the lessons, and learn from them.

▶ Be true to yourself, and don't change to please others.

▶ Engage in your own self-development, and appreciate how it can change your life.

▶ Make sure you have some alone-time to recharge, discover who you really are and ground yourself.

▶ Perfection is a belief you're conditioned to accept but is unattainable.

▶ Seek help if you're struggling with depression, anxiety or panic attacks. There's no shame in admitting you're not coping with life. You don't have to put up a front of 'I'm okay' or 'I'm fine'. Reach out to others, and you will be surprised by the support you receive.

▶ Your family dynamics has no bearing on who you are as a person. Just because you're an only child doesn't mean you're different or that you don't fit in. You're special and unique.

▶ Know that other people's perceptions of you, and their hurtful words, don't define you as a person but are a reflection of who they are. Allow them to work through their judgements without it impacting you.

▶ Life is a journey. Accept that you're on your own path, which will be different from everyone else's.

▶ Be your own best friend, and love yourself for who you truly are.

▶ Have fun. Be wild and adventurous.

▶ Discover what lights up your world, and follow your passion.

Why is a holistic approach to life so important?

Because the mind, body and spirit are interconnected, they form a holistic approach to life.

It's important to understand that if one part of this equation isn't in balance, it ultimately affects the rest in some way.

To achieve ultimate health and wellbeing, you must be mindful of what's going on in all areas of your life.

What are you passionate about?

▶ Experiencing the freedom to do what I love, having fun, being adventurous and free spirited, and travelling the world

▶ Experiencing the magic and mysteries of life and all it has to offer

▶ Studying how the mind works and the way it influences behaviour

▶ Caring deeply about people through love and connection

▶ Appreciating the impact of values and belief systems in society

▶ Studying communication types and how perception influences the outcomes of everyday life

▶ Understanding that the people who come into your life are there to teach you. Everyone has a story to tell and a lesson to share, and it's through these experiences that a bond is created with those who cross your path

▶ Knowing that people come into your life for a reason, a season or a lifetime, and that it's all part of life's journey.

"Follow your passion. It will lead you to your purpose."
~ Oprah Winfrey

Do you utilise alternative therapies?

Yes. I've become open to all forms of alternative therapies. They led me to study and become a practitioner of Australian Bush Flower Essences. I regularly treat and use the essences for myself, my family and my clients by customising the drops specifically for each physical or emotional condition. It's vibrational, energetic medicine.

My training into the world of shamanism and becoming a Shamanka (a female shaman) has been a journey of learning and awakening the healing wisdom into our present-day consciousness. Shamanism isn't a religion or a new-age trend. It's an ancient medicine that involves the practice of putting the body into a state where it's able to heal itself. There are many different techniques that can be used, including energy from crystals. It's simply one of the oldest healing techniques known to mankind, dating back thousands of years.

I cherish my ability to assist in healing others with ancient wisdom.

What is your approach to life?

My approach to life is my *7 Steps to Personal Freedom* system.

1. Give yourself permission to start

Setting the intention to do things differently is the most important step you can take.

Your life can be so busy that you might not know where to start. Each day you have thousands of thought processes going through your mind, and it can feel overwhelming to make the necessary changes.

If the way you're presently living isn't working anymore, the solution is as simple as telling yourself, *I give myself permission to change*. This gives your unconscious mind a direct command that it's okay to try something new. Changing your mindset and perceptions gives you the ability to achieve anything.

2. Overcome life obstacles

There are many obstacles that can stop you from achieving your goals and make you feel trapped and overwhelmed.

It doesn't matter if the obstacle is a mental, emotional or physical issue. If you break the problem down into small steps, it will become easier to achieve. And when you find solutions, it will encourage and challenge you to come up with ways to think differently and overcome the bigger problems.

Instead of looking at what seems impossible, look at what you can do to achieve a purposeful life.

3. Find your authentic self

Finding your authentic self will make you happier, more energised and at peace with who you are. People wear many masks in everyday life and hide behind them as a way of seeking acceptance and approval, or see them as a representation of who they think they are.

You were born to be a unique human being, but you're conditioned from a young age, through societal values and belief systems, that you need to conform to be accepted by others.

By removing the masks and being true to yourself, you'll let go of your own perfectionism and the expectations and judgments of others, and be able to face your fears.

This is where your real transformation starts. The question to ask yourself is, *What mask do I hide behind, and how can I discover who the authentic me is?*

Through my holistic approach to my life coaching sessions, I help people remove their masks to reveal their shadow values and perceptions that are holding them back from reaching their true potential.

4. Create a bucket list

When I felt like I couldn't achieve my goals, I wrote a list of everything I wanted to experience. Some call it a bucket list. The process is quite empowering.

Your list doesn't have to be filled with goals that are complicated, expensive or difficult to achieve. It's more about challenging yourself to create new life experiences. You won't know what's possible until you expand your thinking.

There were two books I used to challenge my thinking and create my bucket list: *Things To Do Now That You're 40* by Rebecca Hall and *Things To Do Now That You're 50* by Robert Allen. They include ways to think creatively, how to set ambitions and goals and nurturing activities to refresh the soul.

By achieving many small goals along the way, and expanding your mind as to what's possible, you'll change your perception and thought processes.

Think big. Anything is possible.

5. Practice love and gratitude

The Beatles sang, 'All you need is love', and it's true! Love is all you need. In fact, there was a study done at Harvard University that proved it. To be loved and needed provides you with a sense of purpose.

You need to understand that you're perfectly imperfect, so having tolerance, compassion, respect and empathy towards others is important. Sharing your life with friends and companions is essential. To love others, and be loved, is what life is all about.

Connecting, bonding and learning from your connections, and the community that can be created by them, is vital to your wellbeing.

Practising daily gratitude means getting more of what you want to experience in life. You might have heard of the book and movie, *The Secret*, that's all about the endless possibilities that are available if you learn how to feel grateful for what you have. I follow this principle daily and truly believe it's been a pivotal part of many of my most amazing life experiences. Ask, and you shall receive.

6. Find your passion

When you're passionate about life, it sets you on fire. You need to sink into your heart space and ask yourself what lights you up and makes your heart sing.

Everyday life will seem easier when you do what you love, which will give you meaning and purpose. Even though it may be scary, get out of your comfort zone to explore what that could be. The rewards will change your life immensely and bring you joy.

7. Achieve freedom

This includes:

❖ Loving yourself unconditionally and acknowledging who you want to be

❖ Removing limitations and taking action to explore what's possible

❖ Becoming your authentic self and creating the life you want

❖ Making decisions that are best for you and loving others without conditions

❖ Doing what you love

❖ Travelling and experiencing the world and all it has to offer

❖ Being happy and reaching your true potential

❖ Continuing to dream about what you want your life to be

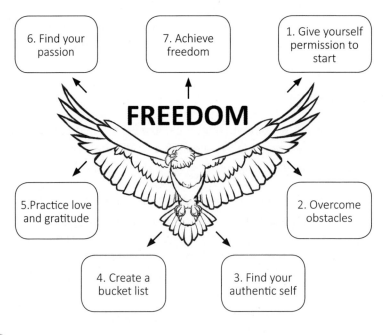

Do you have any parting words you would like to share?

Live each day as if there's no tomorrow, and always remember...

DO WHAT YOU LOVE, LOVE WHAT YOU DO AND LIVE YOUR LIFE WITH PASSION!

To find out more information, including future women's retreats and holistic life coaching services, visit my website at www.kathymorrison. com.au and _The passionate Travel Tribe_ or find me on Facebook and Instagram.

 To discover more about how _Kathy_ can help you _Elevate Your Wellbeing,_ simply visit www.elevatebooks.com/wellbeing

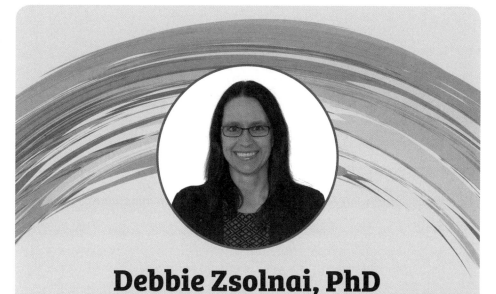

Debbie Zsolnai, PhD

Managing Stress with Mindfulness

Debbie Zsolnai, PhD, is a meditation and mindfulness instructor, author and educator.

She believes that true healing only happens when the root causes of illness are treated and not just their symptoms. Her holistic approach combines multiple natural and complementary methods that work to guide people back to their best self.

In addition to being a practitioner of stress management and its associated illnesses, Debbie empowers people, through education and the sharing of knowledge, to respond to life, rather than react to it.

Debbie is passionate about helping people realise their innate power and potential for self-healing and self-discovery.

Debbie Zsolnai, PhD

Managing Stress with Mindfulness

What got you interested in managing stress with mindfulness?

I became well acquainted with stress while working in the corporate world. In one of my most stressful jobs, where I stayed for twelve years, I often worked seven days a week, eighteen hours a day, trying to meet impossible deadlines. I caught every little bug going around and had no personal or family time.

One day I was sitting onsite at one of my clients, trying to finish up some testing on their system while worrying about the work piling up with another client, when I suddenly began shaking uncontrollably. I thought. *I can't do this. I can't fit it all in*, and I wondered if this was what a nervous breakdown felt like. Shortly after that I ended up in bed for two weeks with a terrible bout of flu. Needless to say, the work was all waiting for me when I got back to work.

This is when I decided enough was enough. I knew there had to be a better way. And there was. By changing my job, as well as my mindset, lifestyle, and routines, I became much happier and able to deal with whatever life threw at me. Now I rarely, if ever, get ill, I'm always happy, and my ability to deal with daily stressors has vastly improved.

What are you passionate about?

I'm passionate about sharing what I've learned, so I can empower people to take their health and healing back into their own hands.

Through the course of my studies, I've learned so much about the link between thoughts and the biology of the body, and how these work together to impact us, right down to our cells, genes and molecules.

 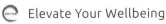

I've learned about the terrible effects stress has on the body, the numerous illnesses it causes and what can be done about it.

I work for an emergency services organisation and get to see firsthand the impact that stress has on people.

What courses have you taken that enabled you to get started or build your business?

I've always had a fascination with understanding what drives people's behaviour, as well as all things metaphysical. I find the link between thoughts, beliefs, mindset and biology riveting.

This is what led me to a degree in psychology, followed by a doctorate in the metaphysical sciences. I'm also working on my energy psychology certification.

I've completed an advanced certificate in teaching meditation and run weekly meditation sessions.

I've also studied Reiki, Emotional Freedom Techniques (EFT), sound healing, colour therapy, aromatherapy, Quantum Touch, energy medicine, mindfulness, epigenetics, neuroplasticity and neuroscience.

What can I say? I love learning.

But even more than that, I love imparting what I learn and empowering others through education and the sharing of knowledge. I want to help people realise their innate power and potential for self-healing and self-discovery. I can't describe the thrill I get from learning something new and sharing it with others. It's gratifying to sit back and watch them respond to life, rather than react to it, and live by design, rather than by default.

What is your approach to healing?

There are four aspects that comprise your health and wellbeing: the mind, spirit, body and emotions. All four need to be integrated, balanced and in harmony when seeking optimum health.

I believe that true healing is only accomplished through treating the cause of the illness, not just the symptoms. I look to combine multiple natural and complementary methods, especially since different approaches work for different people, and there's no *one size fits all*.

When it comes to managing stress, and the associated stress-related illnesses, there are a number of natural tools and remedies that can be utilised. Mindfulness and meditation form just a small part of my overall approach to healing. I also teach about:

- using energy techniques to raise the level of energy, or *qi*, in the body

- how walking barefoot in nature connects you with the earth and promotes healing

- healthy eating and drinking enough water

- the importance of getting enough sleep

- the benefits of exercise, like doing yoga, *tai chi* or *qigong* (a Chinese system of physical exercises and breathing control that's related to *tai chi*)

All of these work together to promote overall wellbeing.

There's also journaling, visualisation, affirmations, social connection, altruism and gratitude, all of which affect your body, right down to gene level.

Additionally, I teach a number of exercises that work to rewire and reprogram your brain, helping to make you less reactive to stress.

What do you think people's greatest barriers are to health and wellbeing?

I think people have forgotten how to slow down and just reconnect with themselves.

How often do you manage to take time out for yourself by maybe going for a nice, slow mindful walk in nature or turning off all of your devices and sitting in quiet contemplation for a while? How about just taking the time to connect with others, face to face, instead of over email or text message?

These days, everyone is so stressed out, so just setting aside a little time for yourself will lead to taking back control of your life.

But although I believe stress is the number one cause of illness today, it hasn't always had a negative connotation.

Do you mean stress can be good?

The relationship between stress and illness is quite complex. A stressful event that causes illness in one person may not cause it in another, as their susceptibility to stress may be different.

Additionally, events must coincide with a wide variety of background factors to manifest as illness, such as coping style, level of social support and personality type.

When confronted by a problem, you need to assess it and determine whether or not you have the resources necessary to deal with it. If you perceive you don't, then you consider yourself under stress. Your method of reacting to these situations makes a difference in regard to your susceptibility to illness and overall health.

Hans Selye, one of the pioneers of the modern study on stress, coined the word *eustress* to define stress that's good or beneficial.

Everyone experiences stress at some point in their life, but it can have beneficial effects. For instance, it can help you develop or learn the necessary skills to cope with, and adapt to, new situations. When the body tolerates stress and uses it to enhance performance or overcome lethargy, it's positive and healthy. However, these beneficial aspects diminish if the stress is ongoing and continuous.

Without stress, you wouldn't be motivated to get out of bed every morning and leave the house to go and work for the things you need.

Stress is negative only when it exceeds your ability to cope and causes physical problems. This harmful stress is called *distress*. The difference in meaning has fallen away, until everyone now thinks of all stress as something negative.

Another difference to understand is between acute and chronic stress.

Acute stress is a response to a stressor of short duration, such as making a speech or taking an exam. Sure, there will be psychosomatic symptoms, such as an upset tummy, or perhaps a headache, but it will also make you feel excited and challenged. And overcoming this acute stressor can make you feel more confident and skilful.

Chronic stress is a response to a stressor that continues for an extended period of time. Examples include jobs in emergency services or law enforcement, caring for a sick child or parent and feeling unqualified to deal with the challenges of your job. If you feel helpless to do anything to change your situation, it could lead to symptoms such as fatigue, sleep disturbances, weight gain and high blood pressure.

Again, it's key to note that the stress won't kill you; it's your reaction to it that will.

How does someone know if they're stressed?

Here are the questions to ask yourself:

- ▶ Do you sometimes struggle to fall asleep at night?

- ▶ Do you find your day just runs away with you, and you can't seem to fit everything in?

- ▶ Do you occasionally feel overwhelmed or irritable?

- ▶ Do you sometimes become snappy with work colleagues or family/friends but don't really know why?

- ▶ Do you sometimes find it hard to concentrate or maintain focus for extended periods?

- ▶ Do you suddenly feel flat or sad but have no idea why?

- ▶ Do you suffer from any physical aches or pains?

- ▶ Do you have a tendency to comfort eat, or perhaps use alcohol or drugs, to try and feel better, deal with pain or just numb out?

- ▶ Do you sometimes feel bored or procrastinate, even though you have so much to accomplish?

- ▶ Do you catch every little bug going around?

- ▶ Do you suffer from overall poor health?

If you answered "yes" to some, or perhaps even all, of these questions, then I think it's safe to say you're suffering from stress.

When is stress bad for you?

Whatever the source of your stress might be, after a while it can make you feel tired and worn out.

When you're stressed out, your thoughts race madly, your heart pounds and your breathing gets shallow. Your muscles tighten, and you struggle to sit still or think straight.

At some point, to try and deal with these reactions, you might numb yourself with mindless eating, alcohol, drugs or endless TV. Or maybe you just push yourself too hard, never taking breaks, and end up wearing yourself out and becoming cranky with those around you.

In the end, you wind up living an unbalanced, unhealthy life, wondering why you're always getting sick and just never feel happy.

What is the stress response?

Your brain's hardwired response is to keep you safe. However, your body isn't always able to differentiate between real and imagined threats.

This stress response has been around for thousands of years. It's what helped your ancestors survive in the days when threats were real. Humans needed to be able to respond rapidly to danger to keep from being attacked or eaten. But this same programmed response isn't good at helping you deal with modern-day stresses.

Let me give you an example.

Imagine two of your ancestors thousands of years ago, Goog and Trang, have decided to head out to find food. They know there's a honeycomb just oozing honey a short distance away, so off they go.

Now, Goog is hyper-alert and paranoid, always jumping at the smallest noise and suspicious of everything. Trang, on the other hand, is easygoing, laughs a lot and is relaxed.

As they make their way to the honey, there's Goog, ever vigilant as she looks for danger. And then there's Trang, smelling the flowers and enjoying the sunlight on her face, not really paying much attention to her surroundings.

They get to the tree safely and are busy eyeing the honeycomb, when Goog spots a Sabre-toothed tiger in the bushes. She immediately screams, drops her bowl and runs, while dear Trang is still looking around in confusion, wondering what all of the commotion is about.

Well, guess who gets eaten?

Yes, it's a silly story, but in evolutionary terms, natural selection favours the paranoid and anxious; those with the ability to quickly get stressed and react with lightning speed.

Now, let's fast forward a hundred-thousand years, and instead of the scene being set out in the wild foraging for food, you're now in your office dealing with rivalries, friction with your colleagues and a demanding boss, all of which raises your stress level.

These kinds of situations don't generally call for physical action, but logistical problem-solving, understanding people's intentions, juggling competing priorities and generally dealing with an ever-changing world in a perpetual state of information overload.

But these are real stressors. Let me give you another scenario.

It's a Sunday afternoon. You've had an amazing morning. You've been out for breakfast with the family, and everything's going well. Even your children are behaving for a change. You're lying peacefully on a picnic blanket at the park, glass of wine in one hand and a book in the other, while hubby keeps an eye on the kids...

Then all of a sudden you realise it's Sunday afternoon, and you have work tomorrow. Back to the grindstone. Maybe you have a big, scary presentation to do, or there's a meeting with your boss, and you have this awful feeling they're going to call you up on your performance or didn't like your last report.

Nothing has changed externally. There's no environmental stressor. This is all going on internally, but now you're experiencing the stress response.

So even without anything happening to turn it on, merely thinking about your problems at work, or what might happen, triggered your emotions and the fight-or-flight response.

When you feel stressed, all of the same biological machinery inside your body turns on as if you were being chased by a tiger.

Your thoughts alone, in your internal mental and emotional environment, have triggered this response not to an actual danger, but a made-up situation in your mind.

Could you explain more about this fight-or-flight response?

When you go into fight-or-flight mode, it hijacks all the resources of your body. Your blood diverts away from your digestive, reproductive and cognitive systems, to your outer limbs. Your muscles tense for action. Your pupils dilate, and your blood sugar, blood pressure and heart rate all rise to free up energy.

Your immune system is suppressed, and as much as eighty percent of the blood in your frontal lobes drains out to feed your muscles, which means it's not a great time for making major decisions.

So by this explanation, you would assume that once the crisis is over, everything goes back to normal, right? Wrong. You then spend hours replaying the scenario over and over, looking at it from all angles, wishing you'd done or said something different. You continue to feel the fury or anxiety that keeps triggering the fight-or-flight response in your body, and it has no way of knowing this threat is all in your mind.

If someone has been stressed for a long time, is it too late for them to reverse the negative effects?

Even if you're already experiencing the negative effects of stress, it's not too late to reverse them.

Until quite recently, it was believed your brain stops growing as you age, and then that's it. If you sustain damage to an area, tough luck. It's never growing back.

But your brain has remarkable abilities to heal and regenerate itself through a process known as *neuroplasticity*. You can literally grow new brain neurons, create positive pathways and enlarge those areas that help you manage stress. By learning which exercises assist you in harnessing the power of your prefrontal cortex, your brain's executive centre, you calm your *amygdala*, so you're able to respond more effectively and mindfully to stress.

Yes, stress is a fact of life, but you don't have to let it overwhelm you and keep you stuck in old ways of thinking and behaving that prevent you from achieving health, happiness and your life goals. You can help keep your prefrontal cortex in charge, so you're less reactive to it.

What is the amygdala?

Your amygdala is an almond-shaped structure right in the middle of your brain that evolved specifically to respond to threats. When it determines there is one, it sounds the alarm. The problem is that the 'threat' can be anything from someone coming at you with a weapon, to a loud crash, to the angry face of someone having a heated conversation with you. Any of these situations can initiate a cascade of physiological changes, with your hormones and neurotransmitters helping prepare you to fight or flee. This is why stress can make you feel wound up and irritable.

The stress response is great if you're facing an acute stressor, such as a guy running towards you with a knife. Before you even have time to think, you react. If you were to stay calm and think things through, you'd probably be a goner.

But it's the chronic stressors you have to worry about.

Mindfulness is just one of a number of tools you can use to manage stress and help put your prefrontal cortex back in charge.

How would you define mindfulness?

Before I give the definition of mindfulness, I'd like to talk about mindlessness.

Have you ever climbed into your car and driven somewhere, and when you reach your destination, you realise you don't remember anything about the journey?

Or perhaps you eat your lunch at your desk at work while reading Facebook posts, and when you reach down to pick up your sandwich for another bite, you discover you've finished it without even realising it?

These are both examples of mindlessness.

Mindlessness is what you do constantly, and mindfulness is what you do rarely.

You listen to people talk while in a mindless state. You watch television in a mindless state. You mindlessly brush your teeth, wash the dishes and take a shower. Basically, almost any repetitive task.

These are all moments lost. Here you were thinking you were living your life, but you weren't even there for most of it. Your mind was off somewhere else.

The antidote to mindlessness is, of course, mindfulness, which is being aware, moment to moment, of what's happening around you.

Mindfulness is a state of being in active and open attention in the present moment. When you're mindful, you observe your thoughts and feelings from a distance and without judgment. You're the observer of the thought, not the reactor to it. Instead of letting life pass you by, your mindfulness allows you to live in the moment, awakened to the experience.

How does someone become mindful?

The great thing about mindfulness is that you can easily incorporate it into your day, because it's your natural state of being. If you have time to breathe, you have time to be mindful.

It's often best to practise mindfulness during those times when you're usually on autopilot mode, like when you're eating, getting dressed or standing in a queue. The opportunities are endless. Here are some mindfulness techniques:

▸ When you're in the shower, focus on the feel of the water running down your back and the smell of the soap or shampoo.

▸ When you're lying in bed, focus on how snug and warm your bed is and how your body feels beneath the blanket, and switch off your thoughts about what might happen tomorrow.

▸ When you're talking to someone, really concentrate on what they're saying instead of thinking about everything you have to do.

▶ Eat and drink mindfully, really noticing and savouring what you're putting into your mouth.

▶ As Thich Nhat Hanh would say, *"Wash the dishes to wash the dishes"*.

By practising mindfulness regularly, you will:

• feel happier

• improve your sleep

• boost your immune system

• enhance your creativity and intuition

• improve your memory and concentration

• enhance your communication skills

• reduce your chances of falling ill

• improve your physical stamina

• increase your motivation

• decrease your stress

In addition, it's even possible for you to lose weight. Cortisol is the body's stress hormone. It's been shown to increase fat accumulation around the waist and hips and is responsible for reduced memory and learning abilities, decreased immune functioning, reduced muscle mass, increased bone loss and interference with cell regeneration.

By reducing your stress, you lower your cortisol, which means an improvement in your overall general health and wellbeing.

Is there any research to support the benefits of mindfulness?

Research has shown that people who practise mindfulness tend to use better coping strategies when in stressful situations, which is due to neurobiological changes in the brain.

By using brain imaging techniques on subjects who'd done an eight-week mindfulness course, neuroscientists were able to observe changes in the 'threat system' of the brain. Specifically, there was a reduction in the reactivity and density of neurons in the amygdala and increased activity in areas of the prefrontal cortex that help to regulate emotions, thereby reducing stress.

Other research into the electrical signals of the brain has shown that ongoing mindfulness practice was associated with increased alpha wave activity, which is linked to relaxation and decreased anxiety.

Furthermore, brain scan technology showed more connections being generated between different areas of the brain, as well as an increase in myelin, a protective nerve tissue essential for healthy brain function.

So mindfulness helps you manage stress, not just because you sat still for a second, but because there are actual beneficial changes in the brain. How cool is that?

Research has shown that mindfulness can lead to:

- better physical health

- improved immune system functioning due to an increased antibody count

- better sleep, weight management and creativity

- improved focus

- managing pain more effectively without the use of painkillers

- quitting bad habits, like smoking

- overall satisfaction and wellbeing

Speaking of painkillers, what makes people medicate with drugs and other substances?

Sure people are stressed...and worried...and anxious...and bored. But hardly anyone is dealing with the root cause. What they usually do is mask the symptoms with medical drugs that make them temporarily feel better, which leads them to think they've dealt with the problem.

You feel emotional pain for the exact same reason you feel physical pain. It acts as a signal that something's wrong that needs attention and fixing. If you're walking down the street, and a sharp stone in your shoe constantly jabs into the sole of your foot, would you rather ask a doctor for a drug to take the pain away or stop and remove the stone?

Drugs just dull the pain, and health spas or vacations make you happy for a limited time. So many people spend a fortune on the 'latest' cure for unhappiness or turn to drugs, alcohol or mindless eating just to try and fill the emptiness inside while numbing their pain.

But everyone holds the key to their own magical pharmacy: the brain.

Your brain is like a dispensary, holding all the healing compounds you need. Everyone is capable of secreting a number of chemicals that can enhance immune function, provide protection from feeling pain or cause the feeling of pleasure. For example, endorphins, the body's natural painkiller, have quite similar effects to morphine.

And the best part? Endorphins are free. So are all the other natural biochemicals secreted by your brain and often consist of the same substances found in prescription drugs. They're also easily assimilated by the targeted organs and systems in doses that won't harm you and don't have all the nasty side effects.

Plus, you can prescribe these for yourself once you know how.

Studies show that meditation, spiritual practice, social connection and goodwill have beneficial effects on every system in the body, but they're rarely publicised.

Meditation measurably improves the body's ability to resist the effects of stress and disease. It can also:

- lower blood pressure

- improve resting heart rate

- reduce the incidence of strokes, heart disease and cancer

- reduce anxiety and depression

- diminish chronic pain

Surely this should be on every doctor's prescription pad, right?

Instead, people use dangerous drugs, either through ignorance or the inability to face the underlying issues.

But surely there's a place for conventional medicine, right?

Well, of course meditation and mindfulness alone aren't going to solve all of your problems and lead to perfect health and wellbeing. Sometimes you do need surgery and the drugs that only doctors can prescribe. What I'm suggesting is that you should be open to exploring other options to healing as well.

There are stories of people who've cured cancer with meditation and visualisation, and while this won't work for everybody, it's certainly worth a shot.

Whatever else you're doing to support yourself, give alternative medicine a try as well. Use every possible resource at your disposal, including conventional and alternative medicine, to support your health and wellbeing.

What are some tools or strategies you would recommend for maintaining a healthy life balance?

There are so many things you could try. What might work well for one person, may not work for another. So try out different options until you find what works for you.

Here's a sampling of some of the tools I teach to get you started:

1. **Practise becoming more mindful**

   Mindfulness gives you a tool you can use when you're in a stressful situation. It helps you turn the lens inwards. Pause and notice your breathing. Don't try and control it. You don't need to change it. Just notice where it is and what it's doing, and sit with it for a while. This switches you out of thinking mode and into sensing mode.

   Try using a mindfulness app. There are a number of free ones you can set to ring periodically throughout your day to remind you to pause and notice how you're feeling. Follow these steps when you hear the reminder:

   ▸ Stop and pay attention to what you're doing

   ▸ Assess how you're feeling

Elevate Your Wellbeing

▸ Get in touch with what you're thinking

▸ Take a few deep breaths, and bring yourself into the present moment

When you're done, carry on with what you were doing. You will soon notice that what you think, affects how you feel. Every single time.

Here's something else you could try. At regular intervals throughout the day, stop and ask yourself the question, "Am I relaxed?", and then follow these steps:

▸ Take a moment to notice how you're sitting and breathing

▸ Adjust your posture if required, or stretch to release any tension in your muscles and body

▸ Take a few deep breaths, and focus on releasing any stress or tension on the out breath

Do this a number of times before carrying on with what you were doing.

2. Start a gratitude journal

Keeping a gratitude journal has changed the lives of so many people. Every day, just write down three or more things you're grateful for, and you will soon reap the benefits.

3. Recognise that you are not your thoughts

Understand that you have thoughts, but you are not your thoughts. You don't have to identify with the stressful voice in your head that's producing them.

4. Notice your tongue

A wonderful tip I learned from one of my teachers, Dawson Church, is to notice what your tongue is doing. Research has shown that when you're stressed, your tongue is usually quite rigid and often pressed up against the roof of your mouth. If you intentionally relax your tongue on the floor of your mouth, it sends a signal to your autonomic nervous system that you're not actually under threat, and your entire body relaxes. Give it a go.

5. Notice your tension

Another trick I love is to notice where you're holding tension in your body. Just focus your attention on it. For example, if you detect that you're tightening your jaw, your shoulders are raised and tight or you're clenching your fist, focus on it, and you will start to release the tension almost immediately, without even having to try.

Is there a significant quote or saying you live by?

There's a great saying that goes, "The essence of Zen is doing one thing at a time".

I love that. It means when you do something, do only that one thing. Don't multitask and think about other stuff you should be working on. Just do it, and move on to the next one...and then the next.

When you're focusing on one task at a time, in the here and now, how could you possibly be stressed?

 To discover more about how *Debbie* can help you *Elevate Your Wellbeing,* simply visit www.elevatebooks.com/wellbeing

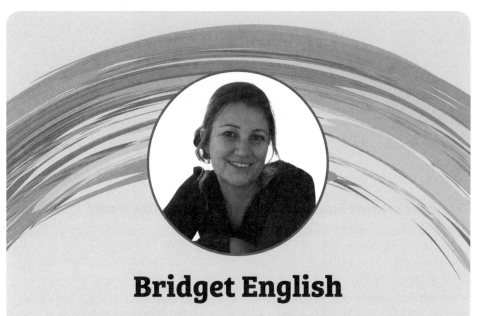

Bridget English

The Healing Powers of Hypnosis

Bridget English is a passionate and experienced hypnotherapist who runs a busy practice in Sydney, Australia. She has a diploma in clinical hypnotherapy, psychotherapy and counselling, and for over a decade has gained extensive hands-on expertise in the industry, specialising in addictions and quit smoking programs.

Bridget is on a mission to awaken people to their limitless potential, so they can pave the way to lasting personal success. Ultimately, she strives to create positive change on a global scale that will perpetuate life transformations for generations to come.

Bridget also volunteers for Lifeline, fights for animal rights and is a devoted mother of two beautiful girls.

Bridget English

The Healing Powers of Hypnosis

What's the one message you wish to share with the world?

I want to share the wonderful healing powers of hypnosis, which I believe is still a mystery to the majority of the population. There are a lot of myths and misconceptions around hypnotherapy, and this means people don't have any real understanding of the way it works as a therapy and how much it can help.

As a practising hypnotherapist, I hope to break the stigma of hypnotherapy and open people's minds to another opportunity for healing, when other methods may have been unhelpful.

How did you discover hypnotherapy?

I had a little part-time reception job while I was living in England, and I often chatted to the people in the waiting room. I remember having a conversation with a lady whose son was upstairs seeing a hypnotherapist.

My first reaction was that I thought hypnosis was only used as a form of entertainment. But then she said that her son had previously been addicted to cocaine and was struggling to overcome depression. She said they'd tried everything to help him recover, and apparently hypnotherapy was her last resort.

She went on to tell me that after her son's first appointment, she checked in on him that night in bed and found him lying on his back sleeping peacefully for the first time in years. It seems that in the past he rarely slept and was always huddled in a foetal position. Seeing him on his back was both emotional and exciting. It gave her a glimmer of hope that he was going to come out of this deep, dark depression and be okay.

They were a football family, and their other son was in the USA playing football professionally. She and her husband had booked flights to visit him, but due to her son's condition, they figured he wouldn't be able to travel with them.

Months later I saw the lady again and asked how her kids were. She said with a big smile on her face, that her son ended up buying a ticket and travelled with them to the USA, because by the time he'd finished his treatments with the hypnotherapist, he was a new man; confident, secure, drug-free and excited about the future.

This was my first introduction to the powers of hypnotherapy and helped me make the decision to change my career path and become a hypnotherapist.

The transformations I've had the pleasure of being a part of have been more rewarding than I could have ever imagined.

How did you become a hypnotherapist?

Due to a relationship breakdown, my two young daughters and I had to move back home to Australia with nothing but the clothes on our backs. After being homeless for a brief period, I found an old rundown house in Parramatta that had been vacant for months. This was probably how we were approved with no references or payslips to show I was actually employed. I used a credit card for the bond, and we found furniture on roadside curbs, charity shops and family and friends. We were in just before Christmas and were truly relieved and grateful.

That New Year's Eve, I decided that things had to change. Though I needed to create a financially secure future for my children, I didn't think I was 'good enough' or 'experienced enough' to even consider opening up a hypnotherapy business, so I advertised on Gumtree that I was available for lawn mowing and cleaning services, as well as airport pick-ups. An Aunty lent me a car that was too old to be eligible for Uber, but it was still reliable.

I would get up all hours of the night to do airport drops for a flat fee of forty dollars one-way. Sometimes it would take up to three hours depending on traffic. The hardest part was keeping the car clean. There were times when I would have a lawn to mow, a house to clean and an airport drop all in one day. If I made a hundred dollars, I would be over the moon!

I believe that in life, everyone is presented with opportunities, and it's up to us to notice and grab onto them. It took me a long time to have the courage to step out of my comfort zone and open up my own practice, but an opportunity arose, and I knew I had to take it.

When I'd completed my hypnotherapy diploma in the UK, the only people I ever used hypnosis on were friends and family. But six months after I'd begun doing odd jobs, an old school friend randomly contacted me and asked what I was up to. When I said I was a hypnotherapist, he invited me to a health and wellbeing festival to promote my hypnotherapy business that didn't actually exist at the time.

After taking the plunge and saying yes, I was forced to make it into a reality. I found an office space, so I could have a location for my 'potential' clients, and also created business cards and a website.

I was told by one of the lecturers at college that only twenty percent of people who study hypnotherapy actually go on to become hypnotherapists. If it weren't for that opportunity, I sometimes wonder if I would still be mowing lawns.

How did you gain the confidence to market to potential clients?

As the festival was drawing closer, and I was feeling overwhelmed, I recorded my own voice to do hypnotherapy on myself, and it worked! To this day, I often do self-hypnosis by recording suggestions and listening to them whenever confidence or other issues come up for me.

What is hypnotherapy?

Hypnotherapy is a natural, simple and relaxing dreamlike state. Once a person is in a trance, they rarely want to come out of it, because it's so euphoric and peaceful. It's the kind of profound relaxation that's hard for them to reach on their own. Some say it's similar to meditation, while others claim it feels like they're floating peacefully. I think it's extremely relaxing, and coming out of a trance feels like waking up from a long, deep and refreshing sleep.

Many people are sceptical or have a negative view of hypnotherapy, because they don't understand how it works and the amount of control they have when in a trance. But they have nothing to worry about, as it's just a form of relaxation, and they're in control at all times.

Could you provide a bit of history behind hypnotherapy?

Most people don't know that hypnotherapy has been around for centuries. There's evidence that hypnosis was used as a form of therapy way back in the 1500s in sleep temples as a way of healing the sick. It's even said that Egyptian priests gave hypnotic suggestions while treating their patients as they stared at metal discs to go into a trance. Some hypnotherapists still use this technique, which is known as *eye fixation*.

The term *hypnotism* was coined in the 1800s by a physician named James Braid, who recognised that the phenomenon of trance had therapeutic value. Braid originally believed that if someone was subjected to a long period of visual fixation on an object, like a watch swinging on a chain, it caused them to enter a deeply relaxed trance state he called *nervous sleep*. This is where the popular image of the hypnotist with the swinging watch comes from. He named this process *neuro-hypnotism*, which he later shortened to hypnotism.

Research suggests that Braid realised verbal suggestion could be used to produce a trance state that significantly increased acceptance to suggestions, but he emphasised that in order for it to be effective, the subject had to be willing to respond.

Generally, hypnotherapists will use the word 'suggestion', which refers to a new idea or direction conveyed to the client. These suggestions are accepted into the unconscious, and a previous behaviour is modified.

How does hypnotherapy work?

The brain is complex and amazing. Without getting into complicated details, I'll just say that within the mind is a conscious and unconscious way of thinking and behaving. The conscious part takes care of the current information needed to carry out your day. You use it to make quick decisions about what to wear, what to do and what to listen to. The unconscious takes care of automatic thoughts, behaviours and habits, and is open and accepting of re-programming old habits and behaviours through hypnosis. The unconscious can also be reprogrammed by consistency. The more you repeat a behaviour, the more it becomes unconscious and therefore automatic.

Why does hypnotherapy work?

Hypnotherapy is a natural state of relaxation. When you're deeply relaxed, the conscious mind is 'asleep' (or distracted), and the unconscious moves to the forefront, which means you're open and ready to receive verbal suggestions. Once the mind has accepted the suggestion, and you awaken from the trance, the body will respond accordingly. You'll have a modified automatic way of behaving, because you've been given a new program that overlays the old one.

However, it's important that you agree to the suggestions. Hypnosis can't make you do something you don't want to, or that's against your values, otherwise the suggestions are rejected. For example, a smoker can't be made into a non-smoker if they don't want to quit. They will always have free choice and can decide to keep smoking regardless of the amount of hypnotherapy they've received.

The conscious mind is the decision maker. The unconscious, or subconscious, does what it's ordered to do. Once a decision has been made, such as 'smoking helps me relax', it's hard to change consciously. Your unconscious will continue running this old program (habit), as it thinks smoking is needed to relax, so it's difficult to quit until the thought is changed using willpower or hypnosis.

What are some of the myths about hypnotherapy?

There are a lot of myths and misconceptions surrounding hypnotherapy. Here are some common ones:

▸ *Myth: you lose control when you're hypnotised*

One of the biggest myths about hypnotherapy is the idea that you automatically lose control during a session. In actual fact, you're in complete control and can't be made to do anything you wouldn't agree to consciously.

This idea is largely influenced by comedic hypnosis stage shows. You've probably been to one and stared in horror as people clucked like a chicken and made a fool of themselves, and you thought, *I don't want to do that!*

Well, let me set your mind at ease and tell you that actual hypnosis is nothing like that.

It's important to understand that it's actually difficult for a hypnotherapist to persuade you to do something out of character, even when you're in a trance.

Stage shows work on the basis that the people who are selected to take part are keen to be involved, are highly suggestible and won't be asked to do anything that's abnormal for them. Anyone who may be uncomfortable with the hypnotist's suggestions, isn't likely to be chosen to go on stage. Also, the techniques used are different from the ones employed for hypnotherapy sessions.

Hypnotherapy is all about putting you in a relaxed state of mind, similar to when you lapse into daydreaming, or the feeling you get just before you fall asleep. You might recall a time you've been driving to work, thinking about something that happened the day before. Then all of a sudden you 'come to' and realise you've driven a great distance without being conscious of it. Or maybe after reading a page of a book, you discover you didn't process it. This is because you were on autopilot and went into a trance. It's completely natural.

A good hypnotherapist can use the heightened suggestibility and reduced inhibitions that come with hypnosis to encourage you to take suggestions on board you may otherwise be less inclined to accept, but this is entirely different from being controlled.

Your hypnotherapist will work with you to overcome your problems, rather than having them be in control of you.

▶ *Myth: Some people can't be hypnotised*

Pretty much anyone can be hypnotised, although the depth of the trance can vary from person to person. This is good news, as it means you have the potential to benefit from hypnotherapy. Anyone can fight or resist hypnosis, and no one can be hypnotised against their will. If you agree to it and allow yourself to sit back and relax, you can be hypnotised.

▸ *Myth: Hypnosis means you're asleep*

People often seem as though they're asleep when they're under hypnosis, but this isn't the case. The depth of trance is so deep and enjoyable, that you enter a dreamlike state.

Your brain is still fully alert and responsive, and some people find that their senses are more heightened than usual.

▸ *Myth: You'll forget everything that happened during hypnotherapy*

Not everyone goes into a deep trance during hypnosis, but if you do, you might not remember some of what happened during the session. This can make you feel as though you must have been asleep or 'out of it'. Though for some people specific suggestions aren't consciously remembered, most recall the feeling of being 'under', as well as the therapist's voice and what they said.

When you're in a deep trance, your conscious mind tends to switch off, while the subconscious mind absorbs all of the suggestions, and this is why you're less inclined to remember. A lot of people only go into a light trance, which is all that's needed for hypnosis, so it means you'll remember the majority of what's said during the session.

▸ *Myth: You may not come out of hypnosis*

Some people are scared they won't come out of a trance, but this isn't possible.

Being in a trance is essentially just a deep form of concentration. You experience trances on a daily basis while watching television or driving long distances, so the concept isn't that unfamiliar.

Your hypnotherapist will be in constant communication with you during your session and will bring you out of the trance at an appropriate time, usually with a simple command to open your eyes.

How does hypnotherapy help people quit smoking?

Smokers are my main clientele. I think it's quite well known how effective hypnosis is with helping people quit. You probably even know someone who was able to give up the habit by using hypnotherapy.

I love hearing from my clients after I've helped them. They're always so elated, because they never thought quitting was achievable after all of their failed attempts.

A recent client who'd been smoking for around forty years said he didn't know how he was going to cope with his anxiety without cigarettes. But when he called me a few days after his session, he said that not only did his anxiety reduce dramatically, he also acted more chilled out in general. In the past he'd felt the need to obsessively clean his house, whereas now he was able to wait. He said there was more to life now that he felt so healthy.

Smoking forces you to take deep breaths. When someone is stressed, they may walk outside to light up a cigarette and wind up feeling more relaxed. It wasn't the cigarette; it was the deep breathing that released endorphins into the body that helped them calm down. A smoker's heart pumps 10,000 more beats per day than a non-smoker, so lighting up that cigarette actually caused more stress to the heart and body.

Hypnosis is completely safe. This is a big plus if you're concerned about the side effects of prescription drugs or nicotine replacement therapy. Though one of those aids could be used as a supplement, studies have shown that you could be successful without them.

The hypnotherapist repeats stop-smoking suggestions while you're in a relaxed state as a way of 'reminding' you of your own motivations to quit. Your unconscious is also reprogrammed to dislike smoking, so when you wake up from the trance, you'll simply feel like you've always been a non-smoker.

Nicotine is one of the most addictive substances known to man, because it tricks the mind into believing it's needed. Therefore, when you decide to stop smoking cold turkey, the mind panics and creates withdrawal symptoms, such as strong urges and cravings, that you most likely give in to. But if you can resist the urge to smoke for as little as one week, you can "beat" the physical addiction. Just as a side note, you should know that the withdrawal isn't painful. It's only an empty or hunger-like feeling, as if you're missing something. After you quit, the habit has been broken, and your mind will stop screaming at you to have a smoke.

Patches, gum and other types of nicotine replacement therapies are often ineffective because they simply prolong the addiction to nicotine. In order for them to be helpful, you must remember to cut back on the amount you use on a daily basis. So once again, it comes down to remembering the motivation and desire.

Why is it so hard to stop smoking?

Smoking is a habit, which means it's hard to break, because you're performing automatic, repetitive behaviours to the point they've become rituals. Your daily life might involve a smoke with a coffee every morning, whenever you get in the car, during breaks at work or when stressed or bored. Human beings love rituals, and it's difficult to change them using willpower alone.

In the case of quitting smoking, hypnosis is highly beneficial, because it allows the therapist to communicate directly with your subconscious mind and confront the habit, thus making the process easier. The hypnotherapist gives suggestions as to why you may want to stop smoking, such as avoiding cancer and heart disease or to stop smelling like an ashtray and feeling like an outcast. They may also use positive outcomes, such as getting more fit and healthy, looking younger, becoming a role model, sleeping better and having more energy.

Hypnosis enables access to the real reason you smoke, which is the mental addiction to nicotine. Quitting doesn't have to be as difficult a process as it appears. It's simply about confronting the habit at its source. Again, the addiction is in your mind, which makes giving it up with hypnotherapy so effective.

Anybody can quit the habit, from the twenty-year-old who only smokes when drinking, to the seventy-five-year-old who smokes two packs a day. It's never too late.

How can people lose weight with hypnotherapy?

Struggling to lose weight is one of the biggest reasons why people turn to hypnotherapy, and if you're currently thinking about using it as a treatment for weight loss, you're probably wondering how it works and the chances for success.

Here are some of the reasons you may be overeating:

▶ **Junk food addiction**

    With junk food being so accessible, cheap and convenient, it can also be addictive. It highlights the pleasure centre in your brain, so you're more inclined to choose the same foods that made you 'feel good' in the past.

▶ **Particular eating issues**

    These can be binge eating, late-night snacking or boredom eating.

▶ **An old pattern of behaviour**

For instance, a lot of women struggle to lose weight after their first child, because of the increase in appetite they experienced while pregnant and breastfeeding. Your hypnotherapist can help you break that pattern.

▶ **As a form of protection**

This can be due to past traumas.

Your hypnotherapist will help you pinpoint why you feel compelled to use food in certain ways, so you can start changing your relationship with it and eat healthier. You may not even realise it prior to starting hypnotherapy treatment, but chances are there are some key reasons why your weight loss goals have been eluding you. Once you know where the problem lies, it's a lot easier to start tackling it through hypnotherapy and to find ways of dealing with emotions and situations, so that food is no longer the answer.

How does hypnotherapy work with drug and alcohol addiction?

It's rare that someone tries a drug with the intent of becoming addicted. Quite often it's for social reasons. They're around friends, people they trust, and they're encouraged or enticed to try it. Unfortunately for some, they become dependent on the feeling the drug or alcohol provides, and they will stop at nothing to get that feeling again and again.

Hypnosis helps you become clean and sober by implanting suggestions into your mind while you're in a trance state and removing the urges, which then makes it easier to avoid the damaging substance. These suggestions may be images of being happy and accomplishing a goal that the substance is making impossible to reach. Or an alarm may go off in your head that tells you *NO* when you see or think of the substance and provides a reminder of the reasons why. It may be an anchor that gives you an unpleasant taste in your mouth when you see or think of the substance. There are many techniques a hypnotherapist can use. It all depends on the client and the nature of the addiction.

Do you have any amazing success stories you'd like to share?

I recently had a client who was addicted to ICE. His life was a mess. He had no job, no money and his family had disowned him. All he had left was his wife, and her entire family had deserted her, because she'd chosen to support her husband through the addiction.

After our first session, he stopped using. I employed a technique that put a guard up in his unconscious mind, so that any time he came into contact with the drug, he would fight the urge and be reminded of the life he wanted to live. He came for a total of five sessions, after which he began the process of turning his life around. It's been over a year, and he now has a great job, most of his family are back in his life and he has a little baby on the way.

Another success story was a young woman who came to me after she was released from hospital. She'd been drinking heavily for years and been admitted to hospital a few times after being found passed out on trains and in shopping centres, but this time it had been life-threatening.

One night, after a concoction of cheap wine and vodka, she'd nearly died by asphyxiation, because she inhaled her vomit, which caused pulmonary aspiration.

After years of counselling and psychology, she decided to try hypnotherapy to remove the urge to drink. On the first session I gave some hypnotic suggestions to build her confidence and strength to remove the thoughts of alcohol from her mind. When she came back for her second appointment, she said that when she got home she realised she'd walked right past the bottle shop without noticing it was there. And while watching TV that night, when she saw someone drinking alcohol, she got a horrible taste in her mouth.

In the next few sessions we worked on her confidence and self-esteem, as well as her motivation for finishing university and mending her relationships with friends and family. It's been eight months now, and she's still free from alcohol.

How does hypnotherapy help with anxiety?

Most people experience some anxiety from time to time. In small doses it can actually be good for you, as it directs adrenalin to enhance your abilities when needed and helps you succeed.

Because it provides an oversupply of adrenaline, runners can use it for quick take-offs, and speakers use it to sound more enthusiastic and generally perform better.

But for some, it's a chronic problem that dominates their life. This can take the form of excessive worrying to the extent that it interferes with day-to-day activities and may lead to a struggle with insomnia, because their mind is constantly racing.

Anxiety can also encourage or exaggerate a range of physical symptoms, such as muscle tension, chronic headaches, and even Irritable Bowel Syndrome (IBS).

This can be distressing and draining, and it can feel as though every day is a constant battle.

Hypnotherapy can be a great way to break this pattern and is becoming more popular as a treatment option. It can also help anxiety sufferers, because it provides the body with a deep state of relaxation that's difficult to create when feeling anxious. Just the act of being in hypnosis brings relief, because it naturally slows your breathing and pulse, and you continue feeling relaxed long after the session is over.

Hypnotherapy can help you regain control and get on top of your anxiety. It taps into a calm and highly relaxed state of mind that's hard to accomplish under normal circumstances, if you're on edge most of the time.

When you're suffering from anxiety, you might be living in a hyperactive state, so your mind doesn't easily switch off, and your negative thoughts race around your brain, making you over-analyse.

Hypnotherapy is most effective in conjunction with cognitive behavioural therapy (CBT) and a hypnotherapist who's also a qualified counsellor. CBT helps when anxiety is caused by your thoughts surrounding certain events, which brings about a reaction in the body. If you can change the way you perceive a situation, you can learn to alter the way you react and feel, and therefore reduce your anxiety.

These are some steps that can help:

▶ *Step 1: Learn relaxation and breathing techniques*

This can take the form of yoga, meditation or mindfulness.

I teach a breathing technique to all my clients who suffer with anxiety that requires you take a deep stomach breath in, and then let it out slowly, as though you're blowing out through a straw. I use this technique often right before public speaking engagements, or any other situation where I might feel anxious.

▶ *Step 2: Exercise*

Exercising helps relieve tension and release calming endorphins. There's evidence that it can greatly reduce anxiety when done at least three times per week.

▶ *Step 3: Question your thinking*

Notice when your thoughts are exaggerated. Begin to monitor them, and when you observe that a thought is negative, try replacing it with a rational one. It might go something like this:

Elevate Your Wellbeing

❖ You're feeling anxious, because your child isn't studying enough.

- Your irrational thought: *He's going to fail. He won't get into university, and his entire academic career is ruined.*

- Your new rational thoughts may be: *He just needs to get back on track. I'll get him a tutor.*

❖ You're feeling anxious, because you haven't heard from your husband all day.

- Your irrational thought: *He's had an accident and is lying dead somewhere.*

- Your new rational thought may be: *He's probably just in a meeting. I would've received a call if something happened.*

The more often you replace fearful thoughts with rational ones, the sooner you'll combat your anxiety. It's a function of your subconscious mind and is supposed to help protect you from fearful situations, so the more you eliminate the thoughts of fearful situations, the more you eliminate unnecessary anxiety.

▶ *Step 4: Learn progressive relaxation*

This is where you focus on your body, part by part, from head to toe or toe to head, and relax each one before moving to the next. This is also helpful in assisting you in drifting off to sleep.

▶ *Step 5: Sleep well*

Make sure you're getting enough sleep, at least seven to eight hours per night. Sleep helps with stress. Situations can seem worse when you're tired.

▶ *Step 6: Eat well*

Make sure you're eating healthy, nutritious food. There's a major connection between diet and wellbeing. You are what you eat, and if you eat crap, you'll feel like crap. Force yourself to cook and eat healthy, and notice the difference in only a short amount of time.

If you're struggling with chronic anxiety and want to break its hold on you, hypnotherapy could be the solution for lasting change. It works a lot better than medication in treating the root cause(s) of your anxiety symptoms and doesn't have any negative side effects. It's a safe and natural way to treat it and could be just what you need to regain control of your mental health.

I had a client who presented with anxiety, which lead to paranoid thoughts about his health. Every time he felt a twitch, he thought he was going to have a heart attack or a stroke. Once the anxiety was relieved, so were his negative thoughts.

Do you have any final words to share?

I hope this chapter has given you some insight regarding the healing powers of hypnosis and how it can reverse unhelpful habits and behaviours, and that one day you choose to give it a go to help transform your life!

 To discover more about how *Bridget* can help you *Elevate Your Wellbeing,* simply visit www.elevatebooks.com/wellbeing

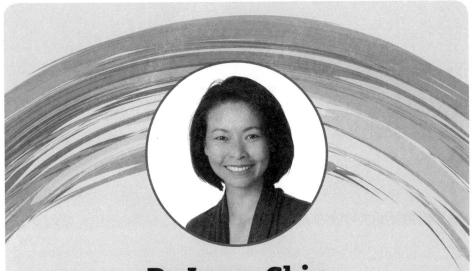

Dr Irene Chin

Finding Joy in Your Pain

Dr Irene Chin is a chiropractor, health coach and teacher. While pursuing her studies, she researched the effects of chronic stress, which gained her a PhD from the University of Sydney, where she's taught for twelve years.

In 2006, she established a holistic and wellness-based chiropractic practice, where she goes beyond alleviating her clients' pain to help them reach their true health potential. She also loves assisting families to become the best versions of themselves and live great big lives.

Dr Irene is certified in the Neuro Emotional Technique (NET), which she marries with gentle low-force chiropractic adjustments, to bring about life-altering changes for her clients.

In addition to being a clinician, Irene is an advocate for sustainability and environmental health.

Dr Irene Chin

Finding Joy in Your Pain

What inspired you to be a chiropractor?

As long as I can remember, I've always wanted to be in a career where I could help people. Traditionally, that has always meant studying medicine. The human body fascinated me, so off I went to university to study medical science. But then during my third year, a friend invited me to a chiropractic philosophy lecture. What I learned there changed my life.

I was reminded that the body has a remarkable ability to heal itself, and health comes from within. For example, if you have a cut on your finger and you put a bandaid on it, does the bandaid heal the wound? No. It keeps the wound clean, so your body can heal from the inside out.

Your body's innate intelligence is expressed through your nervous system, which consists of your brain, spinal cord and the nerves in your body. If your brain and nerves can communicate clearly by relaying appropriate information to and from the rest of your body, it will ultimately function properly and support you as you enjoy life. All your body needs is the right environment with no interference, and that's where chiropractic comes in.

Spinal malalignment (subluxation) can cause nerve interference, which leads to a lack of proper organ function and results in eventual ill health. Because the spinal column is the message highway between the brain and the cells and organs in your body, nerve interferences in the form of irritation, rubbing or pinching, can cause havoc.

What I learned was that chiropractic adjustments remove nerve interference by restoring proper spinal alignment and function, so you can be at your best. No drugging or cutting parts out of the body is necessary. A chiropractor just enhances the intelligence within the body that's already there to heal. That was the lightbulb moment that changed my career path overnight.

How are you currently making a difference in people's lives?

I'm blessed to be in a career where I can make a difference, and I love that what I do is gentle and non-invasive.

Apart from assisting people through my clinical work, I spend quite a bit of my time educating the public on various health subjects, such as the importance of maintaining good spinal health and the impact of thoughts and emotions on their physical wellbeing.

I'm inspired every day by the changes I see in my clients, but there are times I do catch myself taking these changes for granted. I think in society, there are such high expectations to get results instantly, that people (including me) forget to stop and observe the miracle of the healing process.

A few examples of these everyday miracles include:

▸ Aiding a pregnant mum in turning a breeched baby, so she could have a natural birth

▸ Helping a baby sleep and feed better

▸ Witnessing a child's self-esteem increase as their reading and learning abilities improve with treatment

▸ Assisting those who suffer from pain to function and move again, so they can get back to doing what they love

- ▶ Helping students and executives think clearer, so they can excel

- ▶ Guiding athletes to achieve their performance or competition goals

What are you passionate about?

I'm passionate about helping people improve their quality of life and discover what's holding them back. Nothing gives me more joy than making a difference in my clients' lives naturally, without any drugs or surgery.

I especially love working alongside families with children, because I believe if they learn great health habits at an early age, they're more likely to be healthier adults.

Statistics show there's currently an increase in asthma, childhood obesity, and neck and back pain from the upswing in technology usage. Also, depression and anxiety rates, along with doctors prescribing medication for these issues, have soared over the last twenty-five years [1, 2]

There has never been a more critical time than now to focus on the health and wellbeing of families to cultivate a happier and healthier society.

Why don't people make their health a priority, and why is it important to maintain good health?

Good health, happiness and life satisfaction are all linked. According to the World Health Organisation, health isn't just about an absence of disease or illness, it's a state of complete physical, mental and social wellbeing [3].

Staying healthy isn't hard, but it takes work. In my experience, many people don't consider health a priority until disease and illness set in, sometimes to the point where the loss of health may be irreversible. I really hate seeing people suffer, especially when I know it can be prevented.

You can maintain your health by looking after what you have rather than trying to retrieve what's lost. If you acquire all the money in the world, but don't have your health, how can you enjoy it? So it makes good sense to look after yourself.

How does someone go from being well to getting sick?

Stress is a major precursor to sickness. A demanding, modern-day lifestyle, technology dependence and changes in food production and farming, have contributed to the increase of stress in the body.

Even though people have a high capacity to handle stress, if the accumulation overpowers the body's ability to cope, it will start breaking down, and illness can result. This might manifest as:

- headaches

- back pain

- gut issues

- diabetes

- difficulty breathing

- cardiovascular issues

- decreased immune system

- hormonal problems

- insomnia

- depression

- fatigue

Is all stress bad?

No. There's good and bad stress. The good stress, otherwise known as *eustress*, is manageable, because it's usually short-term and can lead to growth and enhancement. Examples include exercise, preparing for a speech and doing something new. The bad stress, or *distress*, is uncontrollable, prolonged, overwhelming and destructive.

Distress can be grouped into three categories:

1. **Physical stress**

   What you do to your body and the physical impact.

2. **Mental stress**

   Your emotional state and how you think.

3. **Chemical stress**

   What you eat, drink, breathe in and expose your body to.

Let's have a look at a few examples of these stressors:

Physical Stressors	Mental Stressors	Chemical Stressors
• Falls and injuries	• Divorce	• Drugs or medication
• Car accidents	• Job loss	• Processed food
• Repetitive strain	• Relationship problems	• Too much sugar
• Bad posture	• Financial difficulties	• Household chemicals
• Lack of exercise	• Death of loved ones	• Pollution
• Lack of rest	• Abuse or neglect	• Pesticides
		• Cosmetics and body products
		• Dehydration

If you're suffering from an illness, or just aren't feeling at your best, I would encourage you to use the above table to do an audit of the life stressors you've experienced within the past twelve months. It can be quite an eye opener! The longer the list, or the more intense the stressors, the more likely you're heading towards ill health and its symptoms. But don't stress out. Let it be a lesson of awareness. Once you know, you can do something about it.

What is pain?

In developed countries, pain is one of the most common reasons people consult their physician. Pain is a perception, meaning it comes from your brain rather than your body. For example, if you place your hand on a hot stove, the sensory nerves send messages to your brain via your spinal cord and brainstem. The brain then processes this information, and if the intensity of the signals reaches the pain threshold, pain perception is triggered, and the unpleasant feeling comes into the forefront of your consciousness, shouting, "Ouch! Mayday!"

Pain isn't just an unpleasant sensory experience associated with actual or potential tissue damage. It also triggers emotional responses [4]. Everyone has a different pain threshold and experience that's influenced by attitudes, beliefs and cultural and social factors. This means that two people with the same pain condition may have two entirely different pain experiences.

Let me take the above example of touching the hot stove. After immediately removing their hand, one person may respond by keeping quiet to deal with the pain, while another might cry and be quite dramatic about it. Have you ever observed such a difference in your world?

Is all pain bad?

Most people will say that all pain is bad, mainly because it's most unpleasant, so the first instinct is to get rid of it. But if you were to have a magic wand to get rid of the pain receptors in your body and not perceive pain, would that be a good thing? Absolutely not! Pain is the body's alarm bell, warning you that something is wrong. It's letting you know that you need to pay attention to what's happening, before more damage is done. Most people have busy minds, so this warning signal is useful in gaining your attention. Pain is crucial, as it's there to protect you.

What makes people medicate with drugs and other substances?

Whether it's physical or emotional pain, aversion to discomfort has a lot to do with dependence on medication. People will focus on the symptoms and seek to remove them as quickly as possible, rather than finding out the cause. This response is instinctive, but it leads away from regaining health.

According to the National Institute of Health, painkillers and sedatives are the two most commonly abused prescription drugs [5]. They activate the reward regions in the brain by increasing dopamine neurotransmitter levels, which results in the pleasure and relief of dysphoria.

Think about it. When was the last time you experienced pain or discomfort? For instance, a headache? Were you tempted to reach for that painkiller to feel better? If your answer is yes, you're not alone. A U.S. federal study reported that prescription painkillers are more widely used than tobacco [6]. In Australia, the consumption of the common opioid-based painkillers such as codeine, morphine and oxycodone, have quadrupled in just over a decade [7].

Here's the tragic news: apparently an aversion to discomfort isn't just causing a high usage of drugs, it's also killing people. A 2011 report from the Centers for Disease Control stated that "Overdoses of prescription painkillers have more than tripled in 20 years, leading to 14,800 deaths in the United States in 2008" [8].

There have been numerous high-profile personalities, including actor Heath Ledger and the singer, Prince, whose deaths were linked to prescription drug complications. All medications, including over-the-counter drugs, need to be considered as dangerous, and caution should be exercised. Too many people are popping pills without an awareness of the consequences.

While seeking comfort in the short term is fine, behaving this way over and over won't serve you and is unhealthy in the long run.

Why are people so averse to pain and discomfort?

Because it's unpleasant, and the human brain is geared towards comfort and pleasure. It's also a survival mechanism. For example, when you were a child, and your parents told you not to touch that sharp object so you wouldn't hurt yourself, it didn't stop you from doing it. The discomfort (pain) made you avoid doing it again. Avoidance of pain provides boundaries and protects you as you venture out into the world. This is a healthy response.

However, severe pain aversion isn't healthy. Neither is an excessive tolerance of it. Avoid being a hypochondriac or an extreme daredevil, so you can have a long and healthy life.

What's a healthier approach to dealing with pain?

The best way is to be proactive and look after yourself when you're well. However, if you're in a place where you're experiencing physical or emotional pain, don't freak out and numb it. When discomfort sets in, it's much healthier to respond rather than avoid it. Imagine how much better it would be if you were able to face it head on and learn and evolve from it. Here are a few steps to confront, and ultimately grow from your discomfort, that I call A.W.A.R.E:

1. **A**sk the right questions

    Ask yourself, *"What are the causes of my symptom(s)?"* Use the Stress Table to list the physical, emotional and chemical stressors in your life.

2. **W**elcome responsibility

   Own it. Be honest with yourself about what role you played in experiencing this pain. There are no judgements, just observations.

3. **A**ssess your emotions

   Identify if you're feeling:

   - fearful

   - anxious

   - angry

   - overwhelmed

   - discouraged

   - hopeless

   - out of control

   - insecure

   - vulnerable

   - self-conscious

   Again, there are no judgements, just observations.

4. **R**ealise the lesson

   Be grateful for your lessons, even when experiencing pain. Physiologically, being in a state of fear increases sensitivity to pain. Being in a state of gratitude eliminates it and increases the sense of wellbeing.

5.   **E**mbrace the learning and grow

Taking a step back and understanding what you've learned and how you've grown from the experience, will help you overcome it.

How can people live up to their potential?

Human nature is reactive. People want to find the easy way in and out. But behaving this way utilises the 'primitive' part of the brain, like in animals. Going above reaction requires thought, questioning, learning and creativity, which are processed in the 'higher' brain centre, or the cerebral cortex.

When you imagine, create and try something new, it activates your cerebral cortex. When you're fearful or reacting to pleasure and pain, you're activating your primitive brain centre.

Humans have a relatively larger cerebral cortex than animals. In fact, it's overdeveloped and accounts for eighty percent of the total brain mass, which is related to higher cognitive abilities than the other larger-brained mammals [9].

While this might be comforting to know, you're probably aware that most people don't make full use of their brain capacity. I'm not talking about the myth that we only use ten percent of our brain. This is about utilising more of your cerebral cortex, which is related to learning, questioning, and creating, in order to live up to your full potential and lead a more purpose-filled life, rather than a reactive one.

It's important to be conscious of your thoughts, because your actions follow. You can create the future you want by thinking creatively and imagining what could be, as opposed to reacting to what's right in front of you.

> "I think, therefore I am."
>
> ~René Descartes

Have you ever experienced extreme pain in your life? If so, how did you overcome it?

I can't say I've ever suffered extreme physical pain, but I've definitely suffered my fair share of deep, traumatic, emotional pain. In the space of five years, I experienced the loss of a set of twins due to complications during pregnancy, the death of my partner, who was the father of the twins, and subsequently finding love again, only to have my partner leave me after nine months of marriage.

I had blow after blow of emotional trauma within a short period of time. When the pregnancy failed, and my partner passed away a couple of years later, I responded by shutting down and blocking my emotional pain.

Yes, I cried and grieved, but my approach was to toughen up and soldier on. I didn't even take any time off work. On many occasions, I would wind up an emotional mess, reacting to memory triggers, especially when I saw pregnant and new mums.

It was then that I discovered the Neuro Emotional Technique (NET), pioneered by a genius of a chiropractor named Dr Scott Walker. It helped me make peace with my past and freed me from the emotional triggers due to my losses.

However, the separation from my newlywed husband just two years later, broke me. It had to be one of the darkest times in my life. I had difficulty getting out of bed, and there was a heavy feeling, like a lead blanket pressing on me, making it hard to breathe.

I've always considered myself strong-minded and tough, so it was like watching a vulnerable stranger. I remember the pain of loss and rejection as I wailed uncontrollably into my pillow. But it wasn't only about my marriage separation. It was the entire past five years of loss that came crashing down on me. I didn't like this emotional hurt and mess or know how to cope with it, so I did what I knew.

First, I got out of bed and went to work. I used what I had, which is my skill to help others. My work and routine were lifesavers. If I didn't have that, I would have remained in bed feeling sorry for myself.

Second, I sat in the pain. For some innate reason, I knew this time I needed to do more than 'heal' from the trauma, so I could feel better. I had to accept the vulnerability of acknowledging the pain and learning from it, no matter how difficult it was. I wanted to get to a place where I took responsibility rather than blaming everyone else, and to be grateful for the lesson, no matter how painful the process. Most importantly, I wanted to remain vulnerable and soften my heart, rather than being the 'toughened up' me I'd been previously.

It took over a year of counselling and NET sessions for me to evolve and grow. During that time, I also made an effort to experience self-love by looking after my body with exercise, weekly chiropractic care and eating nutritiously. I've learned to embrace that vulnerable stranger and came to realise I'm more complete with her. My experience has led me to being more resilient and insightful, and I'm happy with the person I am today. I'm now grateful for discomfort and challenges, as I see them as triggers for self-awareness and growth.

What is NET?

The Neuro Emotional Technique (NET), was originally developed to help chiropractors address recurring spinal subluxations (nerve interference) and the associated physical symptoms that have partial emotional overlay. It's a mind-body technique that finds and removes neurological imbalances related to the physiology of unresolved stress.

NET is a tool that can help improve many behavioural and physical conditions, but it's important to note that the technique doesn't cure or heal the patient. Rather, it removes blocks to the natural vitality of the body by 'allowing' it to repair itself naturally. For more information, please go to *https://www.netmindbody.com*

How do you stay on track with your health and wellbeing?

I've developed a more holistic approach to my wellbeing by making a habit of starting the year with goals written in my journal. I review them every quarter to keep me on track and have found it so effective, that I started running annual goal-setting workshops.

My goals are organised into seven categories:

1. Spiritual health

This is about understanding my place and purpose in life. Though there are various methods of exploring spiritual health, including meditation, spending time in nature or through faith and religion, for me it's about learning to be still, praying and spending time with God.

Being still has always been a struggle for me. My mind is ever racing, and I'm always going and doing. Am I great at being still now? Hell, no! However, flagging it means that I'm conscious and working towards it. Success might take years, but I'm a lot more still now than, let's say, ten years ago!

2. Intellectual health

This is about being inquisitive and engaging in learning new ideas and activities. I know that expanding my mind helps me become well-rounded and healthier.

I love being challenged. My yearly calendar is dotted with continuing chiropractic education seminars. However, I would also like to make sure I attend at least one personal growth seminar a year. I've found that the more I learn, the less I realise I know. It's a humbling experience.

3. Emotional health

This is about checking in with how I'm feeling. Am I relaxed and on top of things, or am I overwhelmed and stressed?

Keeping my feelings in check helps me be responsible for my emotional health, rather than pointing fingers at others. Maintaining a healthy emotional life is one of the keys to happiness.

I don't know about you, but like many people, I'm my own harshest critic. However, I've noticed this kind of thinking goes hand in hand with being harsh with the closest people in my life.

After stumbling upon NET, I've discovered much about why I react this way and learnt to embrace emotional triggers as a chance to learn more about myself. Now, if something gets my goat, I'll ask myself, *Why am I reacting to this?* Being okay with vulnerability has allowed me to grow. The result is life-changing.

In my chiropractic office, I've found that marrying NET with traditional chiropractic care creates fantastic results for my clients, especially for those with recurring ailments. Whether I'm conscious or not about the emotional stressors, stuck emotions can wreak havoc on my health. Resolving it doesn't just take the stress off my body, it also gives me so much freedom and joy!

4. Physical health

This involves maintaining a healthy body. It's asking myself, *What can I do to help me be physically healthier?* It might be moving my body and exercising, eating vegetables and fruit and cutting out sugar, getting more sleep or receiving preventative health care.

Looking after your physical health is the key to having a long and healthy life. Just like with any habit, cultivating a good physical health routine takes time and effort, but it gets easier with practice.

One physical health goal I find challenging is getting seven to eight hours of sleep a night. For many years, I've thought sleeping a waste of time. Crazy, huh? I've always been driven to accomplish a lot, and I was hooked on the feeling of success that comes from it. Sleeping an average of five to six hours a night had become a habit. I didn't know my limitations when it came to pushing my body, until I experienced difficulty breathing and developed heart palpitations. After numerous blood and physical tests came back negative, I realised there was only one thing that would resolve the symptoms: more rest and sleep!

I also have a regime when it comes to eating: The 80/20 rule. Eighty percent of the time I eat clean, which means fresh veggies, fruits and a small portion of meat, while for the other twenty percent, I'm more relaxed. For instance, my twenty percent looks like good dark chocolate, hot chips, coffee and wine.

5. Financial health

Financial stress can be detrimental to your health and relationships, so it pays to plan.

Taking the steps to plan for my financial future means saving, budgeting and managing my resources, while thinking and planning for my financial health.

To be honest with you, money was never my focus or priority in life. Before setting financial goals, I wouldn't have much to show. Don't get me wrong, I was a pretty good saver, but that's about it. I had no plans besides using it for holidays or buying that awesome outfit.

Intellectual pursuits were up there in the ranking of importance, as I've spent thirteen years at university obtaining three degrees. But I questioned why so many of my friends had more money security than I did, especially those in the finance industry.

I remember quizzing a financially successful friend who's way ahead of the game in terms of finances. When I asked her how she became so savvy, she said it wasn't rocket science. When I tried to make excuses, like, "But I don't know anything about money and investment" she said, "Ask questions, seek advice and learn about how to budget and invest. You become good at whatever you focus on."

Since making financial health one of my goals, I've actively sought advice, and I can definitely notice the results.

6. Career health

I believe that my enrichment and personal satisfaction can be obtained through my work. Why would I want to spend so many hours a day doing something I hate?

I'm blessed with a career that I love and find fulfilling. Nevertheless, I still re-examine my job satisfaction regularly to avoid complacency.

When reviewing my career, I ask myself these questions:

▸ Do I still enjoy my job?

▸ How can I add more value to my clients?

▸ Do I need to upskill?

▸ Am I happy with my work-life balance?

▸ Have I taken enough holidays?

I love what I do, but in the past, especially when I was starting my practice, I never prioritised taking holidays, and soon enough, it started to affect my health and focus. What this taught me is that to have longevity and enjoyment in my career, I need to pace myself. My career is not a sprint, it's a marathon. So now I make sure annual holidays are scheduled into my calendar. The more rested I am, the better the practitioner I am.

7. **Social and relationship health**

This relates to developing my relationships and my participation in the community.

Humans are social creatures, and research has shown that isolation is a stress that can lead to difficulty sleeping, decreased healing, chronic illnesses and increased mortality [10]. It's essential for your health and wellbeing to develop and engage in nurturing relationships, as well as having strong social networks that give you support and guidance, especially in times of stress.

Since I'm guilty of being 'too busy' to catch up with family and friends, I've had to diarise my catch-ups in person or on the phone, or time will just slip by, and my relationship with family and friends will suffer.

I've found that being mindful in all these seven areas allowed me to grow and be on purpose in life.

Another key in balancing my quest for wellbeing is having an attitude of gratitude. I've learned to cultivate a habit of being grateful for what I have right now, even if my situation is difficult.

Having a spirit of gratefulness for the now and thankfulness of what the future may bring, disperses stress as I continue to work towards my health goals. In some instances, being grateful for my right now, made me realise I didn't need or want some of the things I had on my goal list. Ultimately, gratitude, married with goal setting, helps me create a more joyful and contented life.

None of these approaches came naturally to me. For example, to create a habit of being grateful, I took a photo of something I'm grateful for each day for 365 days. Yes, that was a year-long project, but all it took was consistency, and it worked! You can check it out on my Instagram, *@irene365grateful*.

Do you have any last words of encouragement?

I hope you've been encouraged. Let all of your discomforts be lessons and an opportunity for growth and wholeness. Be grateful for the now, and set goals to create a joyous and healthy future. Take courage, and shine in your imperfections.

My favourite singer, Leonard Cohen, summarised it perfectly in the chorus of the song 'The Anthem':

Ring the bells that still can ring

Forget your perfect offering

There is a crack in everything

That's how the light gets in.

 To discover more about how *Irene* can help you *Elevate Your Wellbeing,* simply visit www.elevatebooks.com/wellbeing

References:
1. Anxiety and Depression Association of America. Facts and Statistics. (https://adaa.org/about-adaa/press-room/facts-statistics)
2. https://www.theguardian.com/news/2013/nov/20/mental-health-antidepressants-global-trends
3. World Health Organisation definition of Health
4. Definition derived from International Association for the Study of Pain.
5. https://www.drugabuse.gov/sites/default/files/rx_drugs_placemat_508c_10052011.pdf
6. National Survey on Drug Use and Health https://www.samhsa.gov/data/sites/default/files/NSDUH-FFR2-2015/NSDUH-FFR2-2015.htm
7. Berterame, S., Erthal, J., et al. (2016). Use of and barriers to access to opioid analgesics: a worldwide, regional, and national study. The Lancet. Volume 387:10028, p1644–1656, 16 April.
8. https://www.cdc.gov/drugoverdose/pdf/policyimpact-prescriptionpainkillerod-a.pdf
9. Suzana Herculano-Houzel (2009) The Human Brain in Numbers: A Linearly Scaled-up Primate Brain. Frontiers in Human Neuroscience. 3: 31
10. Cacioppo, J. T., Hawkley, L. C., Norman, G. J. and Berntson, G. G. (2011), Social isolation Annals of the New York Academy of Sciences, 1231: 17–22.

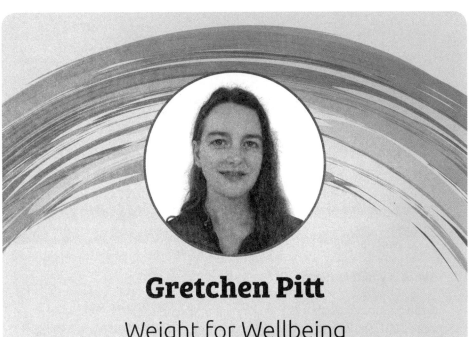

Gretchen Pitt
Weight for Wellbeing

Gretchen Pitt is a trainer, coach, speaker and author. She holds a Bachelor of Arts degree with majors in psychology and history, and is a certified Scrum professional who's worked in the software development industry for over ten years utilising the Agile methodology.

Gretchen enjoys working with others to deliver results. She's had significant weight loss success with the low carbohydrate, high fat (LCHF) meal plan that she incorporated into her exercise and mindfulness techniques and enjoys sharing her knowledge with others to help them regain and maintain a healthy lifestyle.

Gretchen Pitt

Weight for Wellbeing

What is the one message you wish to share with the world?

Foods can harm and foods can heal. Fat is not the enemy.

What is your big WHY?

Growing up, I was always the skinny girl. It didn't matter what I ate, I never put on weight. I also had an extreme sweet tooth. My morning breakfast was about a cup of sugar piled onto cold Weetbix. I could eat a can of condensed milk in one sitting. And come Easter, my siblings and I would wait until there were price reductions on the Easter eggs and buy them up big time, only for them to be gone in less than a week. It was absolutely not healthy, but I never showed any signs of this affecting me.

In my teenage years I began an unhealthy relationship with eating. At one stage I had braces for around two years. Hard and chewy foods hurt to eat and would either get stuck in the braces or my teeth. I began bringing cartons of custard to school for my lunch and wasn't really eating the right nutrients. I was a fussy eater and ate slowly, which meant I would choose quick and easy food rather than anything substantial.

Hitting my twenties meant being away from home and cooking for myself, so I'd opt for healthy meals such as vegetable stir fries and lentil curries, as well as experimenting with other healthy choices.

I was still skinny. I even joined a gym with the express aim of gaining weight, but I wasn't successful. Then a certain man came into my life who I fell head over heels for. He wanted to help fatten me up a little, so he would buy me takeaway food such as burgers and KFC. I also thought he was helping me out by driving me everywhere when previously I would walk. A year later, with this sedentary, junk-food-laden life, I began to put on weight. Though I wasn't eating junk food every day, I was eating a lot more than I had previously.

Fast forward six years, and I'd put on 25 kgs. It was somewhat gradual, so when I stepped on the scales and saw 75 kgs staring back at me on my 162 cm frame, it was a wakeup call. My partner had also put on some weight, so we decided to try eating healthy and avoid fast food. Trouble for me was I did most of the cooking, and he either didn't offer to help or would suggest the quick alternative instead.

Around this time, my father was getting sicker. He had hereditary liver problems that severely affected his life, and my mum had to quit her job to be his fulltime carer. When a compatible liver became available, he underwent a successful liver transplant. This was a stressful time for the family and grew even moreso, when about six months later, my mother was diagnosed with advanced bowel cancer. She'd had to cancel a test a year earlier, as she wanted to travel with my dad to the specialist and could only organise another appointment a year later when it was detected.

My mum was always conscious of her own health and tried to eat well based on dietary guidelines. In a bid to reduce her cholesterol, so that she wouldn't suffer heart attacks like her own mother, she would have the recommended bran and other fibre-filled foods. However, I believe this diet may have exacerbated her condition by causing inflammation to her intestinal tract.

Despite an operation to remove the cancer, it was too late. It had already spread to her liver. My dad offered to have part of his new liver donated to her, but the doctors refused to do the transplant, so she was left with chemotherapy. This didn't stop it, and she passed away in February 2008.

She was the heart and soul of our family, and we all felt lost without her. Then six months later, my partner decided he wasn't in love with me anymore and broke up with me. I was alone, depressed and overweight. I tipped the scales at 80 kgs and knew something needed to change with my lifestyle, but I wasn't sure how to get started.

I began walking for about an hour a day and also eating low fat meals. I did lose some weight but couldn't seem to get below 65 kgs. Disappointment led to old habits creeping back, though I did try more strenuous exercise, getting meals delivered, soup diets and other failed attempts to shift the weight over a period of years.

I then discovered a low carbohydrate, high fat (LCHF) way of eating. I really had to research this thoroughly before I decided to try it out, as it went against the conventional wisdom that going low fat was the way to lose fat. At first I did have some success, however I still couldn't budge the weight I needed to lose. Fast forward to 2016. My father passed away, which caused a lot of stress in my life. I then started not paying too much attention to what I was eating and wound up at 80 kgs again, back where I'd started and just as unhappy.

I decided I needed to do something about this, as I was not going to die as young as my parents had, so I started again reading up on LCHF eating and realised some of the mistakes I'd made. I also changed my mindset to focus on healing my body, so I could lose the weight. In the end I was able to lose 25 kgs in nine months and have kept it off. I now want to share this knowledge with others, so they can also regain their health and wellbeing.

What are you passionate about?

I'm passionate about helping people, which has been an ongoing theme in my work life. I was once asked why I was working as a software business analyst, and I told them that I enjoy getting to the bottom of people's problems and helping them find a solution, to which they replied, "Why are you working in software, then?"

I still think that having software that provides a solution to a problem is a good enough reason to build it, but this also extends to helping people learn and grow. I'm not here to tell people what to do but rather to make suggestions based on the knowledge I've accumulated and point them in the right direction. Then I step back and let them take the necessary steps on their own.

I want people to get empowered, which comes from acquiring knowledge, and I really love sharing what I know to help others.

What's the biggest mistake people make in the area of low carbohydrate, high fat eating?

Eating too much fat. When you're following this program, you need to only eat enough fat to be 'fat adapted', so that your body will then start attacking your own fat. I made this mistake when I first started to eat LCHF. I overdosed on cream and berries and stalled my weight loss, as I was having too much fat after becoming fat adapted.

To be fat adapted, or in ketosis, means your body is using fat as an energy source rather than carbohydrates in the form of glucose. While your body does need some glucose to function, it's not necessary to have it in your diet, as the body will convert the amount of glucose you need from eating lower amounts of carbohydrates and protein.

Getting to fat adaption does require switching to higher amounts of fat than you would normally eat, while at the same time reducing your net carbs to 50 g a day (20 g if following Keto). You then should slightly reduce the amount of fat you have per day once your body is fat adapted.

There are a couple of ways that you can measure if you're in ketosis, which means your body is consuming fat and converting it to ketones, an alternate energy source to sugars. Ketones are produced by the liver from fat and are used by the body as an energy source when there's a lower amount of glucose. The amount of glucose your body needs is produced by the body, so there's no need for extra consumption. One way to measure if your body is in ketosis is to use keto sticks, which are similar to insulin testing. The way I knew was that I listened to my body. Once I stayed fuller for a longer period of time, I knew I'd become fat adapted.

How did you become interested in low carbohydrate, high fat eating?

I'd tried so many different methods to lose weight, including low fat eating, detoxes, infrared saunas and exercise. Nothing worked. I kept sneaking in chocolates and cakes. I did manage to reduce sugar in my tea from three teaspoons to a half a teaspoon. Then one day I happened across a Facebook post from Christine Cronau that eating fat can help you lose fat. At first I thought it was impossible, but I was intrigued by the idea, so I decided to look into it further.

What I learned was that you can lose weight by eating fat, but there are a couple of conditions:

1. You need to reduce the amount of carbohydrates, such as anything made from grains, potatoes and foods that are high in sugar, including some fruits and vegetables.

2. It needs to be a healthy fat, which includes certain nuts, olive oil, avocados, butter and animal fats.

What is your approach to your health?

Health is more than one element. It encompasses the body, mind and spirit. If you neglect one of these, it can impact your overall health and wellbeing.

So when switching to LCHF, don't just focus on food. It's also about nourishing your body and mind.

There are three phases when it comes to eating LCHF:

Each phase will require you to adjust your food intake by looking at your macro nutrients, which are carbohydrates, protein and fat. Don't rush it. There's no quick fix for years of poor diet.

Phase One: Getting Fat Adapted

This is probably the hardest phase, because it's about changing your mindset and relationship with food and gaining an understanding as to what nutrition should mean and how it applies to your bodily cues. It's also about gaining an understanding of what causes you to eat bad foods and how you can avoid or deal with those situations in a constructive way by replacing bad habits with better ones.

Phase Two: Fat Burning

This is when your body is using fat as fuel. The aim of this phase is to ensure that your body fat, along with dietary fat, are both being used as a fuel source.

Everyone is different, and getting to this point can take anywhere from two to six weeks, or in some cases even longer. One of the key indicators that you're in this phase is when you recognise you're not as hungry any more.

Your body will change, though the scale won't always reflect this. As you feed your body the food it really needs, your bones will become denser, and your muscles more developed. These are heavier than fat cells, so while you might lose a dress size, it's possible you won't see a decrease in kilos. However, if you keep going with the program, it will happen.

Phase Three: Maintenance

This is where you reach your goal shape and continue to eat LCHF. You will no longer have the body fat to burn, so you will need to increase your dietary fat and possibly adjust your protein. You're able to eat more carbohydrates, however they should be the good kind. Don't go back to your old habits of eating breads, pastas or sugar. Think vegetables that are higher in carbohydrates such as carrots, beetroot or the occasional sweet potato. If you really want the full health benefits, then only eat them occasionally.

During each phase, look at other aspects of your health. I believe that exercise plays a vital role in health and wellbeing, but exercise by itself won't assist with weight loss for some people. I've been there and done that. But what it will do is help tone your body and reduce stress, if done properly, while also allowing for those happy endorphins to work. You don't need to go running for miles. In fact, if you only did yoga a couple of times a week, it will help. Finding an exercise you enjoy is vital, because if it's a chore, you will always find a way out of doing it.

Other helpful habits you'll want to incorporate, include looking after your GUT health, finding time to relax and reflect and getting enough sleep.

During my coaching sessions, I include ways to incorporate healthy habits into your life. Taking one step at a time helps with not being on information overload. My aim is to ensure understanding of this lifestyle, rather than just telling you what to eat, as it's the only way you'll reap the full benefits.

Based on your experience, what's the most helpful tip you could give?

Listen to your body. Don't disregard any symptoms. Eat when you're hungry, drink when you're thirsty and make sure you get the rest you need every day.

Why is mindset important?

You need to have a clear reason why you would want to follow this way of eating and not just follow it because someone told you to or take on their motivations as your own. It needs to be for you. This way of life can be hard to maintain if you don't set your mind to commit to it. There are a lot of obstacles that will trip you up, such as social occasions like going out to eat, work functions and parties. You need to be strong. People who have the best of intentions may insist you eat that slice of birthday cake or try to convince you that just one slice of pizza won't hurt. But if you can prepare yourself mentally for these challenges, you'll be in a better place to continue without falling off the wagon. Remember your reasons when you feel your resolve weakening.

How does someone keep inspired on a daily basis?

Daily inspiration should come from how you're feeling. Once you're fat adapted, you will most likely feel great. Or at least improved.

Step away from the scale. This advice might sound odd, since you've always used it as your measure of success. But though you may initially lose some weight, you might not see a drop for a couple of weeks or even gain a little as your body adjusts to the different way of eating, and you could become discouraged. Rest assured this is normal. I recommend taking body measurements with a tape measure before you begin and also snapping a few photos. Believe me, you will want these.

Then every two weeks, or once a month, weigh yourself and redo the measurements. You'll be able to see progress. A dexa scan, which is an enhanced x-ray machine that measures bone density, is a real bonus. I'm fortunate that the gym I go to has a body scanner, and I was able to track my percentage of body fat decrease once a month over time.

Though the scale may not move, you'll notice your clothes fitting a lot looser and your face getting thinner, especially if you put before and after photos side by side, so take those pictures. My camera shyness stopped me from taking them, and it's the one thing I regret.

Inspiration can also come from others who are following a similar path. Reach out to Facebook groups and follow Instagram or blogs. Many people will gladly share what has worked for them, as well as their tips and recipes.

Is meditation or mindfulness something everyone should practice?

Absolutely. Stress is a major factor. Even if you eat well, you can still come undone by stress. It produces hormones that can put your body in a flight-or-fight mode. If this happens on a continual basis, your body reacts and goes into survival mode. Find ways to take time each day to just pause and reflect, be it a walk in the park, meditating before bed or sitting with a pet. It's a chance for your brain to slow down, and it stops you from focusing on the cause of your stress.

Mindfulness will then spill over to other aspects of your life, such as your dietary habits. Savour your food. Enjoy the flavours. Make time to sit and eat and not always be on the run.

What are some of the ways people create a barrier to losing weight?

One common barrier people create is telling themselves they won't be able to lose weight or settling for their current state of health, because that's what's expected at a certain age. You can limit your success with this kind of self-talk. You need to turn these negative thoughts into positive affirmations, such as "I will lose the weight". Or even better, "I have lost the weight". Keep reinforcing in your mind that you can do this.

I understand what you're going through, because I had convinced myself I was the weight I was supposed to be. Then when I got to my lowest point, I began looking at myself in the mirror and telling myself out loud, "I am healthy and I am slim". I kept repeating this when doubts started creeping in. Eventually it got to the point where this was true, both in my mind and body. I was able to look back once I'd reached my goals and realised, Yes! This is my truth!. At the time it felt like it might take a while, but in the end it happened in the blink of an eye.

Another barrier is letting other people's' negative expectations enter your own thoughts. Not everyone is going to be accepting of your new habits. It goes against the dietary guidelines that have been pushed onto us for so long. But if you arm yourself with knowledge, you'll be better off. You may not convince others, but reminding yourself of why you're doing this will help reinforce that you're doing the right thing for you.

What's the best way to set and achieve goals?

Setting goals is a way of getting to where you want to go. If you want to lose weight, I suggest taking small steps and setting targets along the way. Don't be too aggressive with them. Make them achievable. Celebrate successes and hitting the small goals. Reward yourself with something that will further nourish you, particularly something not food related. Get a massage, go to a movie or buy some clothes.

Don't be too upset if you didn't reach a goal in a certain timeframe. Instead, acknowledge that it didn't happen and then reflect on what you could do to get to that goal in the future. It might mean re-examining what or how you're eating. Determine what other factors may be at play. Don't be discouraged by setbacks. Arm yourself with knowledge, and listen to your body.

When you set a goal, make it specific. It could be that you will drop a dress size by a certain date. Though it's tempting, try and avoid setting it based on a certain weight. You'll find progress could be slow while you're repairing muscle and bone composition, as these are heavier in mass than body fat.

What's your simple formula for health?

Listen to your body. If you're craving something, it may mean you're deficient in a certain nutrient. If you feel sick, then take a look at what foods may have contributed to that feeling.

With LCHF, you eat when you're hungry and stop when you're full. Make time for yourself each day, and get adequate rest.

Is technology helping or hindering us?

When it comes to LCHF, technology can help. There are many apps you can use to track what you're eating. This is great if you're starting out and are not sure how much to eat. There is one caveat: it's much better to use it as a learning device until you know what you're doing, and then stop using it.

Also, social media is a great help in the form of groups and peer support. There are many out there. You may need to pick and choose, as some have strict rules as to what you can post or how they follow LCHF. This way of eating requires individual adjustments, so one size does not fit all. As long as you go in with that attitude, you'll be able to disseminate the good advice from the bad.

 To discover more about how *Gretchen* can help you *Elevate Your Wellbeing*, simply visit www.elevatebooks.com/wellbeing

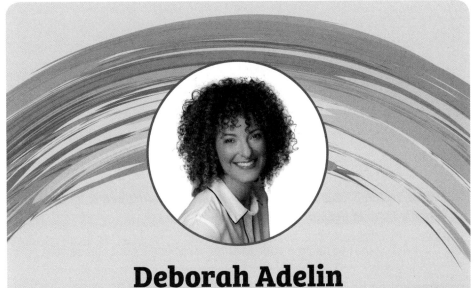

Deborah Adelin

Value Your Values

Deborah Adelin is an author, speaker and lifestyle entrepreneur. She's held a senior leadership role in a BRW Most Innovative Company, as well as managing wellness programs in an aged care organisation and a leading mental health hospital. In addition, she's a qualified life coach who's received training in Acceptance Commitment Therapy (ACT) and Process Communication Method® (PCM).

Deborah has received recognition and an award for her scientific research into the reliability and validity of observational gait analysis, a clinical decision-making tool used globally.

Her transformative vision guides people to defuse and embrace the discomfort that comes from living an expansive life.

Deborah's mission is to help people create a rich, full and meaningful life and align their highest values to daily inspired action.

Deborah Adelin

Value Your Values

What training and accreditations have you participated in that enabled you to get started or build your business?

Over the years, I've had the good fortune of holding a senior leadership role in a BRW most innovative company, as well as managing wellness programs in an aged care organisation and a leading mental health hospital. I hold an honours degree in prosthetics and orthotics, and I'm a qualified life coach and fitness trainer.

I'm humbled to have received recognition and an award for my scientific research into the reliability and validity of observational gait analysis, a clinical decision-making tool. I've also received training in Process Communication Method (PCM) and Acceptance Commitment Therapy (ACT).

My interest in the psychological and physical aspects of wellness and dis-ease led me to spend over twenty years helping leaders, entrepreneurs and mavericks in their field to make a difference. During that time, I founded a total of four organisations across the personal development and sustainability sectors in Australia and Hong Kong.

When I started practising mindfulness to effectively transcend my own deep-seated chronic anxiety and depression, I was surprised by the dramatic results. Over the years I've used mindfulness-based approaches with others and have obtained equally outstanding outcomes.

Currently, I'm fascinated by what goes into having a rich, full and meaningful life. After spending years studying and learning experientially, I want to share this information with as many people as I can.

What is your top tip for someone to elevate their life?

Take action. I'm inspired by the words of Jack Canfield: "You don't have to get it right; you just have to get it started".

Have you had any aha moments that changed everything for you?

Absolutely. Not too long ago, I was struggling to find a career path that really aligned to my essence and reason for being. I knew I wanted to serve humanity and make a tangible difference to people, but I was unclear as to the capacity with which I could make it happen.

Then I made the decision to invest heavily in my education around mindset, wellness and entrepreneurship. I recall the day my mentor helped me clarify my highest values. That's when a monumental mindset shift took place. I liken it to an awakening. I remember feeling like I'd finally given myself permission to become the divine human I was born to be. I felt an immediate sense of relief and an urgency to take inspired action that was aligned to my highest values.

This experience catapulted me into appreciating just how important it is to uncover your highest values. Once I realised the level of clarity I received from such a simple and easy process, I set off on a mission to inspire people to do the same.

Why is it so important to know your highest values?

Values are the compass and torch of life. They guide you towards meaningful action, illuminate your path and bring you back when you wander off track. You can lean on them in times of discomfort. They're a battery pack to supercharge you when things don't go your way and are your enthusiastic best friends who stay by your side along your journey.

If I were to ask you right here, right now, "What are your top three values?, could you list each of them using one word?" Give it a try in the privacy of your own mind.

How did you go? For some, this is easy. The values just roll off the tongue. They are crystal clear and communicated simply. But for others, it's a confronting exercise.

Why?

Well, it's not that you don't have values. It's just that you may not have taken the time to identify them, or known the process to do so for that matter. If this is you, hold yourself kindly, because your values are waiting patiently within you. All you need to do is reach inside, blow the dust off them, bring them into the light and fully own them.

Why is uncovering your values so important to transformation?

Quite simply, values are life's helpers. I say this, because they saved my life. It wasn't too long ago when I had a series of experiences that tested my resilience and self-love. I speak to the greater conscience when I say that most people at some point in their life have what's often termed a 'dark night of the soul'. It's in the darkest hours, during a time of expansive pain, suffering and transformation, where your limits are tested. It may be triggered by the loss of a loved one or relationship, moving to a new place or experiencing sickness or disease. It may also arise from a place of creation, such as the birth of a child, a new relationship or change of lifestyle. It's in this sacred space that you have a choice: be a victim or rise like a phoenix.

In my formative years, I experienced depression, anxiety, a miscarriage and divorce. While going through this pain and suffering, I had feelings of loss, shame, guilt, fear and anger. I came face to face with my shadow values, which helped me understand how I was meeting my needs in both helpful and unhelpful ways. I was also called to answer the existential questions outlined in PCM: "Am I loveable, trustworthy, competent, wanted, acceptable and alive?"

My mind is no different from yours. Many people confront these questions at some stage in life and are in dialogue with them every day.

The greatest lesson I've learned is to fully embrace the experience of the dark night journey, for therein lies great wisdom. Speaking from experience, I can say it's easy to wallow in self-doubt, limiting beliefs and a 'woe is me' attitude.

What I've discovered, through my own life observations, is that uncovering your highest values brings you into alignment with your higher being. In this way, values help you resolve inner conflict by creating a sense of wellbeing and vitality. Living in alignment with your values is transformative.

It's important to note that values can change as you grow. You can test them out, try them on for size, shuffle them around and modify them unapologetically, as many times as you wish. Because it's your life, you can do it your way.

Identifying your highest values is a potent way of clarifying your purpose and your big WHY. I'm often asked if you can live a rich, full and meaningful life if you don't know what your purpose is. To this I say, "Yes!" People put a lot of pressure on themselves to find their one true purpose. I'd like to take the pressure off by saying that just like values, purpose can change at different times in your life, and you can have multiple purposes that can be found *through* living a values-based life.

'Value your values' is a motto I live by.

What are you passionate about?

I'm passionate about living in alignment with my highest values: wellness, communication and connection. They are my companions and guide me through my life journey. I check in with them every day to ensure my actions are congruent. Being an author, speaker and lifestyle entrepreneur, I not only get to live a life aligned to my highest values, I also get to help others do the same. I'm passionate about being a difference maker. I want to help people raise their vibrational frequency, so they can create abundance in all areas of their life, including health and wealth.

What is your big WHY?

Life is full of choices. You have options regarding how you respond to life events. I believe that the key to living a rich, full and meaningful life lies in the ability to observe and become aware of impermanence. Understand that 'this too shall pass'. You are not your story; you are a human living a human life. It's your relationship to these events, and the lessons you learn about humankind, that's the key.

My WHY is to write and speak about mindset, unique self-expression, loving oneself, I am driven to help others by making an impact through my writing and speaking and to leave a legacy for my children and the world.

What is your big WHY?

You are here for a reason. You were born with your own set of DNA that makes you unique. If you overlay that with a distinctive combination of life experiences, you might begin to see just how truly rare and valuable you are. There has never been, and never will be, anyone like you. You're a one-of-a-kind, single-edition human being. This means that the unique way you live your life and contribute to this world is by your design. You are your own architect.

Elevate Your Wellbeing

It is true that as a human collective, everyone travels this life journey together. But quite frankly, you were born by yourself, and you'll leave your body by yourself. That 'dash' in between your birth and death date is really dependent upon how *you* choose to spend it. What I propose is that you use your highest values as the compass to navigate your way to the end of life as you know it. Why? Because life is for *living* every single day. Given that there are twenty-four hours in a day, and a big chunk is dedicated to sleep, there are about sixteen hours left to do something. So what are you using these hours to create? I propose that you consider what I call your '2 WHY', because two whys added together generate an even bigger, more robust WHY.

The first one is all about the reason you want to invest in yourself and your personal development, while the second is about why you want to contribute to the world and how you can help others. You can harness your first why to exponentially grow your second, and vice versa. This ongoing journey of self-actualisation creates a mirroring effect, where the inner and outer work reflect back on one another. This is the stuff that legacy is built on.

How are you currently making a difference in people's lives?

I believe that leading by example is a powerful way to make a difference to others. When you take inspired action, you attract a tribe of like-minded people. I love inspiring people to harness the power of daily inspired actions aligned to their highest values.

Living is full of actions. It's about doing and being. Even seemingly still practices like sleeping and meditating are actions. They are subtle on the outside but immensely powerful on the inside.

It can be said that the quality of the actions you take each day determine the quality of your life. Every action is a step towards an outcome, whether that result is desired or not. Aligning actions to your highest values supercharges them with purpose and vitality.

Not every action you take is pleasurable, easy, simple and comfortable. In fact, when you truly desire something, for example a productive career, relationship or wellness, it takes considered effort and a determined attitude. By learning from your mistakes, and doing repetitive, mindful practices, you will achieve success. Values are there when the going gets tough, because they underpin the grunt work with vitality and meaning. Values-based, active living creates a sense of wellbeing that endures the pain, suffering and discomfort, and is the foundation of living a rich, full and meaningful life.

I'm a big fan of helping people *align actions with values.*

What's your biggest life lesson?

Each day there are life lessons galore. Golden nuggets of wisdom are present in every experience. You get to decide whether you seek to acknowledge, appreciate and harness them or not. My greatest life lesson is realising you are gently, and sometimes not so gently, nudged towards loving yourself.

An example of this is the idea of behavioural repetition. Have you noticed repeating patterns of behaviour in your life? Many people aren't even aware of actions that play on repeat throughout their lives. I liken it to the model of stimuli and response. When 'X' happens in your life, you respond with 'Y'. Many people sense that their behavioural responses are an automatic default mechanism, but when they look more carefully, they realise they often resort to behaviours that are most familiar to them, such as the 'I'm not (fill in the blank) enough' story.

Why do so many people have an 'I'm not enough' story?

Your 'I'm not enough' story can hold you back or keep you stuck.

The brain evolves to keep you safe. This built-in protective mechanism is the reason why humans have survived as a species for so long. Thanks to your brain, you can anticipate and predict events that might jeopardise your safety. Part of the deal, though, is that you come pre-set with the full suite of normal human expressions, including love, curiosity, joy, sadness, fear, anger, guilt, shock and disgust.

Much of society tends to label these states as either good/bad or positive/negative, and reinforce these distinctions through a love affair with 'happy endings'. The by-product is that it skews your perception of these emotions, which results in many people judging two thirds of normal human emotions as bad/negative. It's no wonder humans tend to avoid them or perceive that they're broken!

You've probably noticed how thoughts and feelings appear as if they have a mind of their own. They come and go as they please, and attempting to control them ends up being a frustrating and tiresome task that can often lead to feeling there's something wrong with you. I can assure you there isn't. Everyone is in the same human boat.

So how do you accept that you'll experience all kinds of comfortable and uncomfortable thoughts and feelings but not get controlled by them? What I'm going to suggest may seem counterintuitive at first, so please open your heart and mind and consider another way.

The key here is to understand that you are not your thoughts or feelings. A road is a road, whether it has traffic on it or not. How you respond to thoughts and feelings is a choice. It helps to practise noticing/witnessing the flow of thoughts and feelings that come and go in response to the actions you take in your day-to-day life.

By taking the role of the observer, you will come to accept that everyday living will trigger all types of thoughts and feelings, some comfortable, some not. When you hold onto them too close, you tend to fuse with them. But if you push them away, you could pretend they don't exist, which often leads to unhelpful behaviour like avoidance, distraction or addiction.

Learning to observe your 'I'm not enough' story, and then defusing it using mindful techniques, is a powerful way to wholeheartedly love and accept your whole self just as you are, so you can keep moving and taking daily action on your goals.

Using this approach will allow your thoughts and feelings to come and go like road traffic, so you can live a richer, fuller and more meaningful life.

I stand by the motto, 'love your whole self'.

What's the best way to help people love themselves more?

I'm a firm believer in learning to embrace your unique self-expression. If you consider that you are not your thoughts and feelings, and you can learn mindful practises to soothe yourself and accept the pain, suffering and discomfort that comes from living a human existence, then who are you? Well, you're a one-of-a-kind human with a unique set of values, actioning your life by design. The way in which you express yourself is your domain. You make your own choices.

Are you currently living an authentic, self-expressed life? There's much debate about whether this can be achieved by harnessing strengths or strengthening weaknesses, or both. Whilst everyone is born with some degree of natural 'talent', there are plenty of people who transform their biggest challenges into their greatest strength of self-expression.

For example, many people with dyslexia strengthen their memories and speaking skills as a result of being unable to rely on reading and writing as their primary mode of self-expression. Therein lies the gift: no matter the card you're dealt, everyone has at least one vehicle of self-expression they can use to plant their flag on this earth and say, "I am here".

If you want to be a leader, you need to deliberately practise your unique self-expression. It's the key to turning up the glow in your lighthouse and not only creating a sense of personal wholesomeness, but you also make it easier for your tribe to see you and gravitate towards you. Humans are social creatures, so experiencing authentic self-expression with other like-minded people provides a sense of belonging, which is one of the keys to living a rich, full and meaningful life.

I'm passionate about empowering people to embrace their *unique self-expression*.

Why do you think people hold themselves back from reaching their higher potential?

That's a huge question, and I will attempt to shed some light on a particular aspect of it.

From my anecdotal research, I discovered that many people are uneasy with discomfort. One of the most uncomfortable experiences is fusing yourself to your 'I'm not enough' story. Having been trained in Acceptance and Commitment Therapy (ACT), I can safely say there are many mindful practices you can do to defuse this story, which is a powerful way of strengthening your self-love.

When you come up against roadblocks and discomfort in life that give rise to unpleasant thoughts and feelings, you can use mindfulness-based techniques to change your relationship with them. Appreciating your whole self, and all that makes you unique, enables you to harness your full self-expression and share yourself with the world, aligned with your 2WHY.

In essence, we resemble an ever-expanding pack. What this means is that you can mindfully continue to step in, and step up into, your own sphere of expansion. When you do this, perceived obstacles can be dissolved with an 'I can handle that!' attitude. Glass ceilings are shattered as you continue to expand in resilience and confidence to handle whatever comes your way.

Remember, you are equipped with your values and your willingness to take action, despite the discomfort. You do it your way with your own unique self-expression, all the while loving, honouring and embracing yourself along the way. There's nothing you can't handle. You are unstoppable. Life can, and will, throw all sorts of challenges at you, but you're equipped with the tools to continue to expand. This is what makes a rich, full and meaningful life.

To live an empowered life, remember: *Expansion is empowered living*.

How do signs and signals guide people?

Have you ever noticed that whisper from within? This is your higher being communicating with you. Often you have to keep yourself still to really hear what it's saying. I believe the purpose of this divine wisdom is to support you along your life journey.

But this wisdom isn't always experienced as thoughts and feelings. It communicates to self through a 'knowing', which is a sign of what's best for you in that moment. Often when you don't listen to these whispers, they get a little louder, and then louder again. If you continue to ignore them, they can turn from a gentle tickle with a feather, to a tonne of bricks falling around you.

This is relevant to all areas of your life, including health, relationships and career.

For example, you've been gifted a most miraculous and exquisite vessel to journey this life in. I'm full of wonder and appreciation about just how remarkable the human body is. The truth is that you only have one body to last you a lifetime, and I'm a firm believer in honouring it by using mindful-based practises.

The human body is a divinely intelligent being, in charge of your welfare. It runs your systems without much input from you. It's so brilliant, it can detect early signs of imbalance and dis-ease. It sends signs and signals to alert you to stop, observe and take action to create change. It tells you to move back into a state of homeostasis. Signs and signals are happening all day and night, and it's important to be in an open state where you can receive these messages clearly.

Mindful exercise and stillness, along with nourishing food and high-quality water, are the keys to keeping the channel open, so you can respond to the feathers before they become bricks. While you can't predict how your body may respond to the natural progression of ageing, you can optimise health and wellness each step of the way. I believe that when you focus on wellness-based practises, you create the best conditions for the body to evolve, and in turn create a richer, fuller and more meaningful life.

Remember: *mindful body care widens the channel that your signs and signals flow through.*

How can people uncover their highest values?

I believe in taking inspired action today. To that end, I created the V.A.L.U.E.S. method, with six practical and easy steps to fast-track anyone towards a richer, fuller and more meaningful life.

There's a simple acronym that encapsulates the entire 'VALUES method':

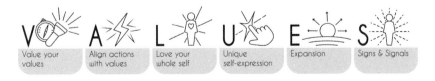

▶ **Value your values**

A dear friend of mine, Benjamin J. Harvey, put together a system known as The Values TRACK®. This next piece of content I would love to share with you comes courtesy of Ben and *Authentic Education*.

The process is all about you and will help you uncover your highest values. There are no wrong or right answers; whatever comes to you, write it down.

In order to dive deep within, it's best to remind yourself that you can freely express your truth, despite thoughts or feelings of fear, shame, guilt or judgment. Give yourself permission to express yourself authentically. Try to complete this exercise as fast as you can. The first response that comes to mind is often your voice. Sometimes by taking too long to respond, you will start to hear other people's answers. The aim is to uncover YOUR unique set of values.

Tip: Values are concepts, more so than feelings.

Respond in full to each question in order, from one to five, with three one-word answers per question. Proceed to question six only when you've completed one through five. Question six requires you to select the one answer from each column that most inspires you. The result of question six is that you now have a list of your five highest values. It's okay if some are repeated.

The Values TRACK®

T	R	A	C	K
1) What do you love to **TALK** about?	2) What do you love to **RESEARCH?**	3) What **ABILITIES** do you love improving?	4) What do you love to **CONTEMPLATE?**	5) What do you **KNOW** a lot about?

6) Select the word from each column above that most inspires you.

Congratulations! You've uncovered, or clarified, your highest values.

- *Are you surprised by your results?*

- *Have you known them all along?*

- *Are you currently living some, or all of them, in your daily life?*

Reminder: You can revisit this exercise as often as you wish, to check in with yourself. It's normal for values to change, so please don't be alarmed if this happens.

▶ **Align actions with values**

Once you've clarified your highest values, you can start pinning or pegging actions to them. A great way to do this is by asking yourself this question:

How can I bring my value to life and breathe action into it?

For example, if wellness, communication and connection were your top three highest values, you might respond like this;

I value wellness so I can:

1. *practice yoga and meditation*

2. *build a business in the wellness industry*

I value communication so I can:

1. *practice ways to communicate my needs to my loved ones*

2. *write a media release article about wellness for the local newspaper*

I value connection so I can:

1. *connect more deeply with myself by recording my daily appreciation/gratitude in a journal*

2. *contact two family members/friends/clients to inquire about their lives*

Hint: Keep in mind that large actions consist of smaller actions. For many, a large action like writing a media release article can seem so overwhelming to do in one go, that it winds up in the too-hard basket.

Actions are best accomplished if they're bite-sized. If they're too small, you can undermine yourself, and if they are too large, you can feel overwhelmed. So if you have a large action, chunk it down into smaller pieces until they're doable whilst stretching yourself. Once you complete an action, ask yourself, *"What's the next 'just-right Goldilocks' action I can take?"*

Reminder: Notice how actions can be orientated around your personal development to meet your needs and fill up your cup, so you're able to cultivate more energy and take actions that make a difference to others. Remember your 2WHY. You can harness the first why, which is your investment in your own personal development, to exponentially grow your second, how you help others.

▶ **Love your whole self**

Here's a way to take a closer look at your 'I'm not _____ enough' story. Take a fresh piece of paper and a pen, and spend thirty minutes filling in the blank. Remember to do your best despite any thoughts or feelings around shame, guilt, judgement or fear. Download all of it onto the paper in front of you.

Once completed, imagine a helium machine and a bucket full of empty balloons. In your mind's eye imagine picking up a balloon the colour of your choosing, and filling it up with helium before attaching one of your 'I'm not enough' stories to it. Let it go, up, up, up and away. Keep going for as long as you want to defuse yourself from the stories that are just words, which are full of air.

▶ **Unique self-expression**

You are a one-of-a-kind human with a unique set of values, actioning your life by design. The way in which you express yourself is unique as well. But too many people seek external approval to be themselves. One way to switch external approval to internal permission is to write a one-thousand reason list. It sounds like a lot, but it can be approached by consistent, daily effort. Try writing fifty words a day for twenty days.

To get started, here are some examples:

1. Why I love myself

2. Why I'm uniquely me

3. Why my unique expression (or what I do) helps others

Hint: Try to push through at least two writing blocks each time you contribute to your list. For the one-percenters, don't stop at one thousand. Keep going! What you're effectively doing is harnessing the brain's ability to create new pathways and connections between pieces of information. Thanks to neuroplasticity and myelination, your brain can continue learning new information and skills via mindful, deliberate practise for as long as you want to.

▶ **Expansion**

When you start something new or deepen your relationship with an existing action, it's common for self-limiting beliefs to bubble to the surface. A way to neutralise these beliefs is to invite them all over for a metaphoric 'cup of tea'. Sit them down at the table and have a chat with them. Take your time to meet and greet each one in turn. Here's an example:

Hello, FEAR! You turn up when I expand myself; I know you like to keep me safe and in the one spot. I appreciate that, but I really am okay. I'm just shining my light in new ways. Thank you, and I love you.

Greet each of them like they're old friends. Remember, their purpose is to keep you on your toes and test your resilience. Harness them to take you to the next level of expansion in life.

Hint: Just like everything you want to get better at, it takes focused practice, so keep at it!

▶ **Signs and signals**

Here's your chance to research, explore and get creative. There are plenty of ways to practise mindful living that keep open the communication between you and your body, so it has a clear channel in which to send you important signs and signals. Setting up a signs and signals 24/7 helpline promotes harmony, healing and graceful aging. Remember that the aim is to respond to the feathers before they become bricks.

Do you have any final thoughts you'd like to share?

Congratulations! Today is an auspicious day. There will never be a younger you or another you. If you're well on your way to creating a rich, full and meaningful life, continue doing what you're doing. If you're not but want to, consider implementing the V.A.L.U.E.S. method as a way of improving your situation. Hold yourself kindly, and appreciate that life is a learning process. Remember that even in your current state, you're extraordinarily valuable to yourself and others!

 To discover more about how *Deborah* can help you *Elevate Your Wellbeing,* simply visit www.elevatebooks.com/wellbeing

Afterword

While you were reading these people's inspiring stories, did you notice something? All of their life experiences were for a purpose, bringing them closer to their goals, relationships and especially the message they were meant to share with the world.

The last page is a blank canvas for you to write the next chapter of your own story about elevating your wellbeing and inspiring others. Every day is a brand-new opportunity to be the author of your destiny.

Next Steps

To support you on your journey to *Elevate Your Wellbeing,* we recommend you take advantage of these resources:

🖥 7 Day Transformation Program

Learn ONE powerful 'Elevate Process' you can use immediately to improve Your Relationships, Health, Finances, Mindset and any other area of your life.

To join this 7-day transformation online program, simply go to: www.elevatebooks.com/you

👥 Connect with the Authors

To discover more about the authors and what they have to teach you, and bonus gifts they are offering visit:
www.elevatebooks.com/wellbeing

🎤 Subscribe to our Podcast

If you'd like to hear the go-to interviews from the authors and be re-inspired, check out: www.elevatebooks.com/podcast

🌐 Visit the Website

To find out more about the Elevate book series, visit: www.elevatebooks.com